FREE Study Skills Videos/DVD Offer

Dear Customer,

Thank you for your purchase from Mometrix! We consider it an honor and a privilege that you have purchased our product and we want to ensure your satisfaction.

As part of our ongoing effort to meet the needs of test takers, we have developed a set of Study Skills Videos that we would like to give you for FREE. These videos cover our *best practices* for getting ready for your exam, from how to use our study materials to how to best prepare for the day of the test.

All that we ask is that you email us with feedback that would describe your experience so far with our product. Good, bad, or indifferent, we want to know what you think!

To get your FREE Study Skills Videos, you can use the **QR code** below, or send us an **email** at studyvideos@mometrix.com with *FREE VIDEOS* in the subject line and the following information in the body of the email:

- The name of the product you purchased.
- Your product rating on a scale of 1-5, with 5 being the highest rating.
- Your feedback. It can be long, short, or anything in between. We just want to know your impressions and experience so far with our product. (Good feedback might include how our study material met your needs and ways we might be able to make it even better. You could highlight features that you found helpful or features that you think we should add.)

If you have any questions or concerns, please don't hesitate to contact me directly.

Thanks again!

Sincerely,

Jay Willis
Vice President
jay.willis@mometrix.com
1-800-673-8175

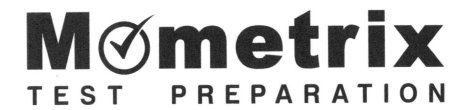

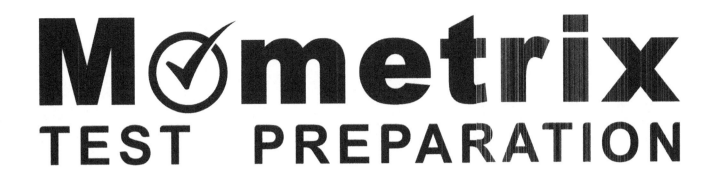

CPC

Exam Preparation 2022 and 2023

Secrets Study Guide for the Professional Coder Certification

Full-Length
Practice Test

Detailed Answer
Explanations

Written and edited by Matthew Bowling

Printed in the United States of America

This paper meets the requirements of ANSI/NISO Z39.48-1992 (Permanence of Paper).

Mometrix offers volume discount pricing to institutions. For more information or a price quote, please contact our sales department at sales@mometrix.com or 888-248-1219.

Mometrix Media LLC is not affiliated with or endorsed by any official testing organization. All organizational and test names are trademarks of their respective owners.

Paperback
ISBN 13: 978-1-5167-2106-1
ISBN 10: 1-5167-2106-3

DEAR FUTURE EXAM SUCCESS STORY

First of all, **THANK YOU** for purchasing Mometrix study materials!

Second, congratulations! You are one of the few determined test-takers who are committed to doing whatever it takes to excel on your exam. **You have come to the right place.** We developed these study materials with one goal in mind: to deliver you the information you need in a format that's concise and easy to use.

In addition to optimizing your guide for the content of the test, we've outlined our recommended steps for breaking down the preparation process into small, attainable goals so you can make sure you stay on track.

We've also analyzed the entire test-taking process, identifying the most common pitfalls and showing how you can overcome them and be ready for any curveball the test throws you.

Standardized testing is one of the biggest obstacles on your road to success, which only increases the importance of doing well in the high-pressure, high-stakes environment of test day. Your results on this test could have a significant impact on your future, and this guide provides the information and practical advice to help you achieve your full potential on test day.

Your success is our success

We would love to hear from you! If you would like to share the story of your exam success or if you have any questions or comments in regard to our products, please contact us at **800-673-8175** or **support@mometrix.com**.

Thanks again for your business and we wish you continued success!

Sincerely,
The Mometrix Test Preparation Team

Need more help? Check out our flashcards at:
http://mometrixflashcards.com/CPC

TABLE OF CONTENTS

Introduction

Thank you for purchasing this resource! You have made the choice to prepare yourself for a test that could have a huge impact on your future, and this guide is designed to help you be fully ready for test day. Obviously, it's important to have a solid understanding of the test material, but you also need to be prepared for the unique environment and stressors of the test, so that you can perform to the best of your abilities.

For this purpose, the first section that appears in this guide is the **Secret Keys**. We've devoted countless hours to meticulously researching what works and what doesn't, and we've boiled down our findings to the five most impactful steps you can take to improve your performance on the test. We start at the beginning with study planning and move through the preparation process, all the way to the testing strategies that will help you get the most out of what you know when you're finally sitting in front of the test.

We recommend that you start preparing for your test as far in advance as possible. However, if you've bought this guide as a last-minute study resource and only have a few days before your test, we recommend that you skip over the first two Secret Keys since they address a long-term study plan.

If you struggle with **test anxiety**, we strongly encourage you to check out our recommendations for how you can overcome it. Test anxiety is a formidable foe, but it can be beaten, and we want to make sure you have the tools you need to defeat it.

Secret Key #1 – Plan Big, Study Small

There's a lot riding on your performance. If you want to ace this test, you're going to need to keep your skills sharp and the material fresh in your mind. You need a plan that lets you review everything you need to know while still fitting in your schedule. We'll break this strategy down into three categories.

Information Organization

Start with the information you already have: the official test outline. From this, you can make a complete list of all the concepts you need to cover before the test. Organize these concepts into groups that can be studied together, and create a list of any related vocabulary you need to learn so you can brush up on any difficult terms. You'll want to keep this vocabulary list handy once you actually start studying since you may need to add to it along the way.

Time Management

Once you have your set of study concepts, decide how to spread them out over the time you have left before the test. Break your study plan into small, clear goals so you have a manageable task for each day and know exactly what you're doing. Then just focus on one small step at a time. When you manage your time this way, you don't need to spend hours at a time studying. Studying a small block of content for a short period each day helps you retain information better and avoid stressing over how much you have left to do. You can relax knowing that you have a plan to cover everything in time. In order for this strategy to be effective though, you have to start studying early and stick to your schedule. Avoid the exhaustion and futility that comes from last-minute cramming!

Study Environment

The environment you study in has a big impact on your learning. Studying in a coffee shop, while probably more enjoyable, is not likely to be as fruitful as studying in a quiet room. It's important to keep distractions to a minimum. You're only planning to study for a short block of time, so make the most of it. Don't pause to check your phone or get up to find a snack. It's also important to **avoid multitasking**. Research has consistently shown that multitasking will make your studying dramatically less effective. Your study area should also be comfortable and well-lit so you don't have the distraction of straining your eyes or sitting on an uncomfortable chair.

 The time of day you study is also important. You want to be rested and alert. Don't wait until just before bedtime. Study when you'll be most likely to comprehend and remember. Even better, if you know what time of day your test will be, set that time aside for study. That way your brain will be used to working on that subject at that specific time and you'll have a better chance of recalling information.

Finally, it can be helpful to team up with others who are studying for the same test. Your actual studying should be done in as isolated an environment as possible, but the work of organizing the information and setting up the study plan can be divided up. In between study sessions, you can discuss with your teammates the concepts that you're all studying and quiz each other on the details. Just be sure that your teammates are as serious about the test as you are. If you find that your study time is being replaced with social time, you might need to find a new team.

2

Secret Key #2 – Make Your Studying Count

You're devoting a lot of time and effort to preparing for this test, so you want to be absolutely certain it will pay off. This means doing more than just reading the content and hoping you can remember it on test day. It's important to make every minute of study count. There are two main areas you can focus on to make your studying count.

Retention

It doesn't matter how much time you study if you can't remember the material. You need to make sure you are retaining the concepts. To check your retention of the information you're learning, try recalling it at later times with minimal prompting. Try carrying around flashcards and glance at one or two from time to time or ask a friend who's also studying for the test to quiz you.

To enhance your retention, look for ways to put the information into practice so that you can apply it rather than simply recalling it. If you're using the information in practical ways, it will be much easier to remember. Similarly, it helps to solidify a concept in your mind if you're not only reading it to yourself but also explaining it to someone else. Ask a friend to let you teach them about a concept you're a little shaky on (or speak aloud to an imaginary audience if necessary). As you try to summarize, define, give examples, and answer your friend's questions, you'll understand the concepts better and they will stay with you longer. Finally, step back for a big picture view and ask yourself how each piece of information fits with the whole subject. When you link the different concepts together and see them working together as a whole, it's easier to remember the individual components.

Finally, practice showing your work on any multi-step problems, even if you're just studying. Writing out each step you take to solve a problem will help solidify the process in your mind, and you'll be more likely to remember it during the test.

Modality

Modality simply refers to the means or method by which you study. Choosing a study modality that fits your own individual learning style is crucial. No two people learn best in exactly the same way, so it's important to know your strengths and use them to your advantage.

For example, if you learn best by visualization, focus on visualizing a concept in your mind and draw an image or a diagram. Try color-coding your notes, illustrating them, or creating symbols that will trigger your mind to recall a learned concept. If you learn best by hearing or discussing information, find a study partner who learns the same way or read aloud to yourself. Think about how to put the information in your own words. Imagine that you are giving a lecture on the topic and record yourself so you can listen to it later.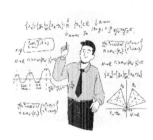

For any learning style, flashcards can be helpful. Organize the information so you can take advantage of spare moments to review. Underline key words or phrases. Use different colors for different categories. Mnemonic devices (such as creating a short list in which every item starts with the same letter) can also help with retention. Find what works best for you and use it to store the information in your mind most effectively and easily.

3

Secret Key #3 – Practice the Right Way

Your success on test day depends not only on how many hours you put into preparing, but also on whether you prepared the right way. It's good to check along the way to see if your studying is paying off. One of the most effective ways to do this is by taking practice tests to evaluate your progress. Practice tests are useful because they show exactly where you need to improve. Every time you take a practice test, pay special attention to these three groups of questions:

- The questions you got wrong
- The questions you had to guess on, even if you guessed right
- The questions you found difficult or slow to work through

This will show you exactly what your weak areas are, and where you need to devote more study time. Ask yourself why each of these questions gave you trouble. Was it because you didn't understand the material? Was it because you didn't remember the vocabulary? Do you need more repetitions on this type of question to build speed and confidence? Dig into those questions and figure out how you can strengthen your weak areas as you go back to review the material.

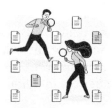 Additionally, many practice tests have a section explaining the answer choices. It can be tempting to read the explanation and think that you now have a good understanding of the concept. However, an explanation likely only covers part of the question's broader context. Even if the explanation makes perfect sense, **go back and investigate** every concept related to the question until you're positive you have a thorough understanding.

As you go along, keep in mind that the practice test is just that: practice. Memorizing these questions and answers will not be very helpful on the actual test because it is unlikely to have any of the same exact questions. If you only know the right answers to the sample questions, you won't be prepared for the real thing. **Study the concepts** until you understand them fully, and then you'll be able to answer any question that shows up on the test.

It's important to wait on the practice tests until you're ready. If you take a test on your first day of study, you may be overwhelmed by the amount of material covered and how much you need to learn. Work up to it gradually.

On test day, you'll need to be prepared for answering questions, managing your time, and using the test-taking strategies you've learned. It's a lot to balance, like a mental marathon that will have a big impact on your future. Like training for a marathon, you'll need to start slowly and work your way up. When test day arrives, you'll be ready.

Start with the strategies you've read in the first two Secret Keys—plan your course and study in the way that works best for you. If you have time, consider using multiple study resources to get different approaches to the same concepts. It can be helpful to see difficult concepts from more than one angle. Then find a good source for practice tests. Many times, the test website will suggest potential study resources or provide sample tests.

Practice Test Strategy

If you're able to find at least three practice tests, we recommend this strategy:

UNTIMED AND OPEN-BOOK PRACTICE

Take the first test with no time constraints and with your notes and study guide handy. Take your time and focus on applying the strategies you've learned.

TIMED AND OPEN-BOOK PRACTICE

Take the second practice test open-book as well, but set a timer and practice pacing yourself to finish in time.

TIMED AND CLOSED-BOOK PRACTICE

Take any other practice tests as if it were test day. Set a timer and put away your study materials. Sit at a table or desk in a quiet room, imagine yourself at the testing center, and answer questions as quickly and accurately as possible.

Keep repeating timed and closed-book tests on a regular basis until you run out of practice tests or it's time for the actual test. Your mind will be ready for the schedule and stress of test day, and you'll be able to focus on recalling the material you've learned.

Secret Key #4 – Pace Yourself

Once you're fully prepared for the material on the test, your biggest challenge on test day will be managing your time. Just knowing that the clock is ticking can make you panic even if you have plenty of time left. Work on pacing yourself so you can build confidence against the time constraints of the exam. Pacing is a difficult skill to master, especially in a high-pressure environment, so **practice is vital**.

Set time expectations for your pace based on how much time is available. For example, if a section has 60 questions and the time limit is 30 minutes, you know you have to average 30 seconds or less per question in order to answer them all. Although 30 seconds is the hard limit, set 25 seconds per question as your goal, so you reserve extra time to spend on harder questions. When you budget extra time for the harder questions, you no longer have any reason to stress when those questions take longer to answer.

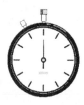

Don't let this time expectation distract you from working through the test at a calm, steady pace, but keep it in mind so you don't spend too much time on any one question. Recognize that taking extra time on one question you don't understand may keep you from answering two that you do understand later in the test. If your time limit for a question is up and you're still not sure of the answer, mark it and move on, and come back to it later if the time and the test format allow. If the testing format doesn't allow you to return to earlier questions, just make an educated guess; then put it out of your mind and move on.

On the easier questions, be careful not to rush. It may seem wise to hurry through them so you have more time for the challenging ones, but it's not worth missing one if you know the concept and just didn't take the time to read the question fully. Work efficiently but make sure you understand the question and have looked at all of the answer choices, since more than one may seem right at first.

Even if you're paying attention to the time, you may find yourself a little behind at some point. You should speed up to get back on track, but do so wisely. Don't panic; just take a few seconds less on each question until you're caught up. Don't guess without thinking, but do look through the answer choices and eliminate any you know are wrong. If you can get down to two choices, it is often worthwhile to guess from those. Once you've chosen an answer, move on and don't dwell on any that you skipped or had to hurry through. If a question was taking too long, chances are it was one of the harder ones, so you weren't as likely to get it right anyway.

On the other hand, if you find yourself getting ahead of schedule, it may be beneficial to slow down a little. The more quickly you work, the more likely you are to make a careless mistake that will affect your score. You've budgeted time for each question, so don't be afraid to spend that time. Practice an efficient but careful pace to get the most out of the time you have.

Secret Key #5 – Have a Plan for Guessing

When you're taking the test, you may find yourself stuck on a question. Some of the answer choices seem better than others, but you don't see the one answer choice that is obviously correct. What do you do?

The scenario described above is very common, yet most test takers have not effectively prepared for it. Developing and practicing a plan for guessing may be one of the single most effective uses of your time as you get ready for the exam.

In developing your plan for guessing, there are three questions to address:

- When should you start the guessing process?
- How should you narrow down the choices?
- Which answer should you choose?

When to Start the Guessing Process

Unless your plan for guessing is to select C every time (which, despite its merits, is not what we recommend), you need to leave yourself enough time to apply your answer elimination strategies. Since you have a limited amount of time for each question, that means that if you're going to give yourself the best shot at guessing correctly, you have to decide quickly whether or not you will guess.

Of course, the best-case scenario is that you don't have to guess at all, so first, see if you can answer the question based on your knowledge of the subject and basic reasoning skills. Focus on the key words in the question and try to jog your memory of related topics. Give yourself a chance to bring the knowledge to mind, but once you realize that you don't have (or you can't access) the knowledge you need to answer the question, it's time to start the guessing process.

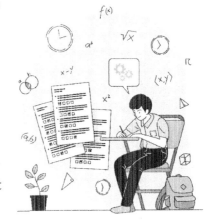

It's almost always better to start the guessing process too early than too late. It only takes a few seconds to remember something and answer the question from knowledge. Carefully eliminating wrong answer choices takes longer. Plus, going through the process of eliminating answer choices can actually help jog your memory.

Summary: Start the guessing process as soon as you decide that you can't answer the question based on your knowledge.

7

How to Narrow Down the Choices

The next chapter in this book (**Test-Taking Strategies**) includes a wide range of strategies for how to approach questions and how to look for answer choices to eliminate. You will definitely want to read those carefully, practice them, and figure out which ones work best for you. Here though, we're going to address a mindset rather than a particular strategy.

Your odds of guessing an answer correctly depend on how many options you are choosing from.

Number of options left	5	4	3	2	1
Odds of guessing correctly	20%	25%	33%	50%	100%

You can see from this chart just how valuable it is to be able to eliminate incorrect answers and make an educated guess, but there are two things that many test takers do that cause them to miss out on the benefits of guessing:

- Accidentally eliminating the correct answer
- Selecting an answer based on an impression

We'll look at the first one here, and the second one in the next section.

To avoid accidentally eliminating the correct answer, we recommend a thought exercise called **the $5 challenge**. In this challenge, you only eliminate an answer choice from contention if you are willing to bet $5 on it being wrong. Why $5? Five dollars is a small but not insignificant amount of money. It's an amount you could afford to lose but wouldn't want to throw away. And while losing

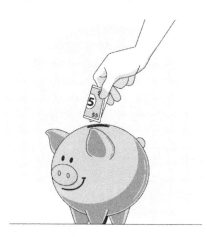

$5 once might not hurt too much, doing it twenty times will set you back $100. In the same way, each small decision you make—eliminating a choice here, guessing on a question there—won't by itself impact your score very much, but when you put them all together, they can make a big difference. By holding each answer choice elimination decision to a higher standard, you can reduce the risk of accidentally eliminating the correct answer.

The $5 challenge can also be applied in a positive sense: If you are willing to bet $5 that an answer choice *is* correct, go ahead and mark it as correct.

Summary: Only eliminate an answer choice if you are willing to bet $5 that it is wrong.

Which Answer to Choose

You're taking the test. You've run into a hard question and decided you'll have to guess. You've eliminated all the answer choices you're willing to bet $5 on. Now you have to pick an answer. Why do we even need to talk about this? Why can't you just pick whichever one you feel like when the time comes?

The answer to these questions is that if you don't come into the test with a plan, you'll rely on your impression to select an answer choice, and if you do that, you risk falling into a trap. The test writers know that everyone who takes their test will be guessing on some of the questions, so they intentionally write wrong answer choices to seem plausible. You still have to pick an answer though, and if the wrong answer choices are designed to look right, how can you ever be sure that you're not falling for their trap? The best solution we've found to this dilemma is to take the decision out of your hands entirely. Here is the process we recommend:

Once you've eliminated any choices that you are confident (willing to bet $5) are wrong, select the first remaining choice as your answer.

Whether you choose to select the first remaining choice, the second, or the last, the important thing is that you use some preselected standard. Using this approach guarantees that you will not be enticed into selecting an answer choice that looks right, because you are not basing your decision on how the answer choices look.

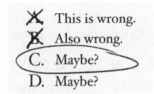

This is not meant to make you question your knowledge. Instead, it is to help you recognize the difference between your knowledge and your impressions. There's a huge difference between thinking an answer is right because of what you know, and thinking an answer is right because it looks or sounds like it should be right.

Summary: To ensure that your selection is appropriately random, make a predetermined selection from among all answer choices you have not eliminated.

Test-Taking Strategies

This section contains a list of test-taking strategies that you may find helpful as you work through the test. By taking what you know and applying logical thought, you can maximize your chances of answering any question correctly!

It is very important to realize that every question is different and every person is different: no single strategy will work on every question, and no single strategy will work for every person. That's why we've included all of them here, so you can try them out and determine which ones work best for different types of questions and which ones work best for you.

Question Strategies

☑ READ CAREFULLY

Read the question and the answer choices carefully. Don't miss the question because you misread the terms. You have plenty of time to read each question thoroughly and make sure you understand what is being asked. Yet a happy medium must be attained, so don't waste too much time. You must read carefully and efficiently.

☑ CONTEXTUAL CLUES

Look for contextual clues. If the question includes a word you are not familiar with, look at the immediate context for some indication of what the word might mean. Contextual clues can often give you all the information you need to decipher the meaning of an unfamiliar word. Even if you can't determine the meaning, you may be able to narrow down the possibilities enough to make a solid guess at the answer to the question.

☑ PREFIXES

If you're having trouble with a word in the question or answer choices, try dissecting it. Take advantage of every clue that the word might include. Prefixes can be a huge help. Usually, they allow you to determine a basic meaning. *Pre-* means before, *post-* means after, *pro-* is positive, *de-* is negative. From prefixes, you can get an idea of the general meaning of the word and try to put it into context.

☑ HEDGE WORDS

Watch out for critical hedge words, such as *likely, may, can, sometimes, often, almost, mostly, usually, generally, rarely,* and *sometimes.* Question writers insert these hedge phrases to cover every possibility. Often an answer choice will be wrong simply because it leaves no room for exception. Be on guard for answer choices that have definitive words such as *exactly* and *always.*

☑ SWITCHBACK WORDS

Stay alert for *switchbacks.* These are the words and phrases frequently used to alert you to shifts in thought. The most common switchback words are *but, although,* and *however.* Others include *nevertheless, on the other hand, even though, while, in spite of, despite,* and *regardless of.* Switchback words are important to catch because they can change the direction of the question or an answer choice.

⊘ FACE VALUE

When in doubt, use common sense. Accept the situation in the problem at face value. Don't read too much into it. These problems will not require you to make wild assumptions. If you have to go beyond creativity and warp time or space in order to have an answer choice fit the question, then you should move on and consider the other answer choices. These are normal problems rooted in reality. The applicable relationship or explanation may not be readily apparent, but it is there for you to figure out. Use your common sense to interpret anything that isn't clear.

Answer Choice Strategies

⊘ ANSWER SELECTION

The most thorough way to pick an answer choice is to identify and eliminate wrong answers until only one is left, then confirm it is the correct answer. Sometimes an answer choice may immediately seem right, but be careful. The test writers will usually put more than one reasonable answer choice on each question, so take a second to read all of them and make sure that the other choices are not equally obvious. As long as you have time left, it is better to read every answer choice than to pick the first one that looks right without checking the others.

⊘ ANSWER CHOICE FAMILIES

An answer choice family consists of two (in rare cases, three) answer choices that are very similar in construction and cannot all be true at the same time. If you see two answer choices that are direct opposites or parallels, one of them is usually the correct answer. For instance, if one answer choice says that quantity x increases and another either says that quantity x decreases (opposite) or says that quantity y increases (parallel), then those answer choices would fall into the same family. An answer choice that doesn't match the construction of the answer choice family is more likely to be incorrect. Most questions will not have answer choice families, but when they do appear, you should be prepared to recognize them.

⊘ ELIMINATE ANSWERS

Eliminate answer choices as soon as you realize they are wrong, but make sure you consider all possibilities. If you are eliminating answer choices and realize that the last one you are left with is also wrong, don't panic. Start over and consider each choice again. There may be something you missed the first time that you will realize on the second pass.

⊘ AVOID FACT TRAPS

Don't be distracted by an answer choice that is factually true but doesn't answer the question. You are looking for the choice that answers the question. Stay focused on what the question is asking for so you don't accidentally pick an answer that is true but incorrect. Always go back to the question and make sure the answer choice you've selected actually answers the question and is not merely a true statement.

⊘ EXTREME STATEMENTS

In general, you should avoid answers that put forth extreme actions as standard practice or proclaim controversial ideas as established fact. An answer choice that states the "process should be used in certain situations, if…" is much more likely to be correct than one that states the "process should be discontinued completely." The first is a calm rational statement and doesn't even make a definitive, uncompromising stance, using a hedge word *if* to provide wiggle room, whereas the second choice is far more extreme.

☑ BENCHMARK

As you read through the answer choices and you come across one that seems to answer the question well, mentally select that answer choice. This is not your final answer, but it's the one that will help you evaluate the other answer choices. The one that you selected is your benchmark or standard for judging each of the other answer choices. Every other answer choice must be compared to your benchmark. That choice is correct until proven otherwise by another answer choice beating it. If you find a better answer, then that one becomes your new benchmark. Once you've decided that no other choice answers the question as well as your benchmark, you have your final answer.

☑ PREDICT THE ANSWER

Before you even start looking at the answer choices, it is often best to try to predict the answer. When you come up with the answer on your own, it is easier to avoid distractions and traps because you will know exactly what to look for. The right answer choice is unlikely to be word-for-word what you came up with, but it should be a close match. Even if you are confident that you have the right answer, you should still take the time to read each option before moving on.

General Strategies

☑ TOUGH QUESTIONS

If you are stumped on a problem or it appears too hard or too difficult, don't waste time. Move on! Remember though, if you can quickly check for obviously incorrect answer choices, your chances of guessing correctly are greatly improved. Before you completely give up, at least try to knock out a couple of possible answers. Eliminate what you can and then guess at the remaining answer choices before moving on.

☑ CHECK YOUR WORK

Since you will probably not know every term listed and the answer to every question, it is important that you get credit for the ones that you do know. Don't miss any questions through careless mistakes. If at all possible, try to take a second to look back over your answer selection and make sure you've selected the correct answer choice and haven't made a costly careless mistake (such as marking an answer choice that you didn't mean to mark). This quick double check should more than pay for itself in caught mistakes for the time it costs.

☑ PACE YOURSELF

It's easy to be overwhelmed when you're looking at a page full of questions; your mind is confused and full of random thoughts, and the clock is ticking down faster than you would like. Calm down and maintain the pace that you have set for yourself. Especially as you get down to the last few minutes of the test, don't let the small numbers on the clock make you panic. As long as you are on track by monitoring your pace, you are guaranteed to have time for each question.

☑ DON'T RUSH

It is very easy to make errors when you are in a hurry. Maintaining a fast pace in answering questions is pointless if it makes you miss questions that you would have gotten right otherwise. Test writers like to include distracting information and wrong answers that seem right. Taking a little extra time to avoid careless mistakes can make all the difference in your test score. Find a pace that allows you to be confident in the answers that you select.

⊘ Keep Moving

Panicking will not help you pass the test, so do your best to stay calm and keep moving. Taking deep breaths and going through the answer elimination steps you practiced can help to break through a stress barrier and keep your pace.

Final Notes

The combination of a solid foundation of content knowledge and the confidence that comes from practicing your plan for applying that knowledge is the key to maximizing your performance on test day. As your foundation of content knowledge is built up and strengthened, you'll find that the strategies included in this chapter become more and more effective in helping you quickly sift through the distractions and traps of the test to isolate the correct answer.

Now that you're preparing to move forward into the test content chapters of this book, be sure to keep your goal in mind. As you read, think about how you will be able to apply this information on the test. If you've already seen sample questions for the test and you have an idea of the question format and style, try to come up with questions of your own that you can answer based on what you're reading. This will give you valuable practice applying your knowledge in the same ways you can expect to on test day.

Good luck and good studying!

Current Procedural Terminology (CPT) Surgical Procedures

Integumentary System

INTEGUMENTARY SYSTEM

The integumentary system is made up primarily of the **skin,** including its multiple layers. Those layers include the **epidermis**, the outermost protective portion of the skin; the **dermis**, the middle layer that consists of connective tissue, hair follicles, sweat glands, and nerve endings; and a layer of **subcutaneous tissue** that connects the outer layers to the muscle underneath and contains blood vessels and nerves. Hair and nails are also considered part of this system.

The integumentary system serves many key functions, including maintaining the body's homeostasis and shape, protecting internal tissues and organs from harm and infection, excreting waste via perspiration, and serving as a sensor for touch, pressure, heat, and cold.

PROCEDURES

Procedures involving the integumentary system are covered by CPT codes **10004** through **19499**, which are divided into related headings and subheadings throughout the section. Procedures in this section cover things that directly involve the skin and certain procedures involving the breasts. In general, this covers procedures including:

- Performing biopsies of skin lesions.
- Removal of skin tags and other lesions.
- Procedures involving fingernails and toenails.
- Introducing substances into the skin.
- Caring for and repairing wounds.
- Skin grafts and skin replacement treatments.
- Destruction of benign and malignant lesions.
- Mohs micrographic surgery.
- Procedures related to mastectomies, breast repair, and breast reconstruction.

Several codes, particularly those related to wound care and repair, are often included in surgical codes in later sections.

SKIN TAGS

Skin tags are small, soft, fleshy and generally benign growths on the skin, often occurring on the eyelids, armpits, neck, in the folds of the groin, underneath breasts, and in other places where the skin folds. Although skin tags are harmless, they can in some cases become irritated and some consider them aesthetically unpleasing. Skin tags are typically removed either with sharp tools (such as scissors or a scalpel), strangulation, electrocauterization, or chemical destruction.

When coding for the removal of skin tags, use code **11200** for the first 15 tags removed, and then use the add-on code **11201** for each 10 tags after the first 15. Fractions of 10 still count toward the use of the add-on code. For example, if a procedure removes 28 skin tags from a patient, the codes used would be 11200 for the first 15, and 11201 twice: once for skin tags 16 through 25 and a second time for the remaining 3 skin tags. Thus, $15 + 10 + 3 = 28$.

WOUND DEBRIDEMENT

Wound debridement is the medical removal of dead, damaged, infected, or otherwise nonviable tissue from an anatomical site. It is typically done to promote healing, prevent the spread of an infection, or remove debris or dead tissue from the area. Debridement can be done surgically, chemically, mechanically (such as hydrotherapy), or by other methods.

When coding wound debridement, take into account the surface area debrided, the depth of the wound that is being debrided, and the anatomical location of the wound being treated. If only a single wound is being debrided, use the code for the deepest level of tissue removed. If there are multiple wounds at differing depths, combine the surface areas of all wounds at the same depth separately from each other. For example, if a 6 cm^2 wound and a 12 cm^2 wound are debrided of subcutaneous tissue while a separate 19 cm^2 wound is debrided to the bone, then only the 6 cm^2 and the 12 cm^2 wounds are added together, not all three.

SUBCUTANEOUS AND ACCESSORY STRUCTURES
FNA BIOPSY

A fine needle aspiration (FNA) biopsy, as defined by CPT, is a biopsy performed when material is aspirated with a fine needle and the cells are examined cytologically. The procedure involves using a thin needle to extract cells from abnormal tissue for analysis to aid in the diagnosis of a disease. This is typically performed on a lesion, cyst, or other type of mass located in or under the skin. An FNA biopsy can be done with or without imaging guidance.

FNA biopsies are covered by codes **10004** through **10012** and **10021**. When selecting the correct code, note what type of imaging guidance (if any) is used, and how many lesions are biopsied. If multiple lesions are biopsied, **add-on codes** (indicated with a "**+**" next to the code number) will be needed in addition to the initial code. For example, two lesions biopsied while using ultrasound would be codes 10005 and 10006. If multiple types of imaging are used during the same session, report the additional codes with the modifier 59. For example, one lesion with no guidance followed by one lesion with fluoroscopic guidance would be listed as 10021, 10007-59.

STANDARD TYPES OF BIOPSIES

CPT lists three types of biopsy, described as follows:

- **Tangential biopsies** are performed with a sharp blade, typically a scalpel, a **curette** (a sharp, hook-like scraping tool), or a flexible blade that cuts or shaves off a shallow sample of the tissue to be analyzed.
- **Punch biopsies** use a hollow cylindrical tool to remove a full-thickness sample of the skin and tissue, similar to taking a core sample from ice or wood. This procedure also includes closing the wound.
- **Incisional biopsies** are when the provider uses a sharp blade to remove a wedge or vertical incision to remove a full-thickness sample of tissue for diagnostic purposes. This procedure also includes closing the wound left behind.

When coding for biopsies, keep track of how many separate biopsies are performed. If different biopsies are all performed on the same lesion, use the primary codes for each different type. If different types of biopsies are performed on different lesions, use the add-on codes instead for each separate lesion mentioned after the first. For example, if three lesions are biopsied, a primary punch biopsy and two incisional biopsies, then the codes would be one 11104 and two 11107s.

16

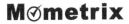

CODING FOR EXCISION PROCEDURES

Codes for excision are initially divided into whether the lesion is **benign** (noncancerous) or **54**of anatomical locations. For example, code 11400 and its associated codes are for a benign lesion on the trunk, legs, or arms.

Finally, when coding for excision, calculate the total diameter of the area being excised. This is done by adding together the lesion's size, plus the margins around it where it is excised. For example, if a 1 cm malignant lesion on a patient's arm is excised with margins of 1.5 cm on each side, add 1 cm + 1.5 cm + 1.5 cm = 4 cm, resulting in the code 11606.

Excision codes include simple closure of the wounds. If an intermediate or complex closure is required, it is coded separately.

NAILS

Procedures in the CPT codebook that directly involve nails and associated structures are covered by codes **11719** through **11765** and include the following:

- Trimming or debridement
- Removal of the actual hard surface of the nail, also known as **avulsion of the nail plate**
- Evacuation of **subungual hematomas,** or bruising or blood under a nail
- Excision of the nail and **nail matrix**, the area where the nail initially grows
- Biopsy of the entire nail
- Repair or reconstruction of the **nail bed,** the tissue underneath the actual hard surface of the nail, including tissue grafts
- Excisions to treat ingrown fingernails or toenails.

PILONIDAL CYSTS

A pilonidal cyst is a type of **cyst,** an abnormal sac filled with fluid or other material, that develops on a person's back, typically located at the base of the sacrum and just above the cleft of the buttocks. Pilonidal cysts typically contain pus, skin debris, and/or hair. They can become inflamed, infected, or painful without treatment. The CPT codes used for procedures to treat pilonidal cysts are **10080** through **10081** and **11770** through **11772**. The codes used depend on whether the cyst is **incised** (cut into) and drained or **excised** (removed) and the status of the cyst at the time of treatment.

WOUND REPAIRS

TYPES

Wound repair codes are used when a wound is closed via **sutures** (sewing the wounds closed), staples, and tissue adhesives, either on their own or in concert. These codes do not apply if a wound is closed using only adhesive strips.

CPT classifies wound repairs into three different types:

- **Simple** repairs are used for superficial wounds, typically only including the epidermis, dermis, or subcutaneous tissue without additional involvement of deeper tissue. Simple repairs involve a single layer of closure, and they often include local anesthesia.
- **Intermediate** repairs include everything listed for simple repairs, but the wound requires layered closure of multiple layers of tissue or extensive cleaning or removal of foreign material. Intermediate repairs can include limited **undermining**, or when the wound extends in multiple directions under the opening but less than the maximum width of the wound's opening.

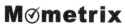

- **Complex** repairs involve wounds that, in addition to everything listed for intermediate repairs, include exposure of bone, cartilage, tendons, or other structures; debridement of wound edges due to trauma; extensive undermining (more than the maximum width of the wound's opening); involvement of the border between the skin and the rims of the ear, nostril, or lip; and/or the placement of retention sutures.

CODING

When selecting the correct wound repair code or codes, first determine the **location** of the wounds being repaired. Codes are grouped by anatomical location within the type of repair, such as simple or complex.

Next, check the **number** of wounds and what types they are. This is important for sequencing codes; the most complicated wound repair is considered to be the primary procedure, and any additional codes are secondary, requiring the use of the modifier 59.

Finally, check the **measurements** of the wounds that are being repaired. Procedures will give the wound sizes in centimeters. If multiple wounds are being repaired, add the total size of all wounds of the same type at the same anatomical location. For example, if a 3 cm and an 8 cm wound on the trunk is being closed with a simple repair and a 6 cm wound on the trunk is being closed with a complex repair, add the two simple wounds together for a total of 11 cm.

SKIN GRAFT PROCEDURES

There are three key factors that must be taken into account when coding skin graft procedures, beginning with identifying the **source** of the graft. Most skin grafts are either **autografts**, which use tissue harvested or cultivated from the patient; or **skin substitutes**, which are from other people, animals, or synthetic skin substitutes. Next, take into account the anatomical **location** of the graft. Like wound repair codes, skin graft codes cover a group of anatomical locations.

Finally, check the **size** of the graft. Grafts are coded with a primary code covering the first 100 cm^2 of a graft, with an add-on code for each additional 100 cm^2 or part thereof. So, for example, an epidermal autograft on the leg that covers 152 cm^2 would use codes 15110 and 15111: 15110 for the first 100 cm^2 and 15111 for the additional 52 cm^2.

This only applies to adults. When dealing with children or infants, code by percentage of body area covered by the graft.

DESTRUCTION

Destruction, in terms of medical procedures, is the ablation or elimination of various defects or lesions via a variety of methods. Methods can include laser surgery, electrical cauterization, extreme cold, chemical removal, or surgical removal. These procedures may include local anesthetic.

When coding destruction procedures, code for whether the procedure is targeting **benign** or **malignant** lesions, as well as the **number or size** of the lesion or lesions being removed. Some codes focus on the number of lesions removed, whereas others (such as 17106 and related codes) focus on the destruction of a single lesion measured in square centimeters.

MOHS MICROGRAPHIC SURGERY

Mohs micrographic surgery is a method used for removing complex or ill-defined skin cancer with histologic examination of the margins. The surgeon acts as both surgeon and pathologist, removing and analyzing the tissue in discrete pieces referred to as **blocks**, which is done in multiple progressively deeper layers called **stages.**

When a provider performs a Mohs surgery, keep track of the number of blocks and the number of stages. Codes **17311** and **17313** are used to code the first **stage**, including the first five blocks, with the associated add-on codes covering additional stages. The add-on code **17315** is used for additional blocks. Therefore, if a Mohs surgery is done on the trunk with four blocks in the first stage and seven blocks in the second, the codes used would be 17313 (first stage), 17314 (second stage with the first five blocks), and 17315 (the additional two blocks on the second stage).

BREASTS
CODES AND PROCEDURES

Procedures that involve the **breast**, here defined as tissues found within the human mammary glands in males and females, are covered by codes **19000** through **19396**. The procedures covered by this section include the following:

- Aspiration of cysts located in the breast
- Biopsies of lesions or abnormal tissue found in the breast
- Excision of abnormal tissues from the breast, milk duct, or nipple
- Introduction of localization devices, primarily for cancer treatment
- Mastectomies
- Breast repair and reconstruction, including the insertion of implanted prosthetics.

Several of these procedures, particularly biopsies and introduction procedures, will include some form of imaging guidance (such as ultrasound or MRI) in the code.

MASTECTOMY PROCEDURES

CPT codes cover three different types of mastectomies, which are differentiated by the type and quantity of tissue removed during the procedure. A **simple partial** mastectomy only removes a portion of the breast tissue from one or both breasts. This is typically the least extreme type of mastectomy.

A **simple complete** mastectomy involves the complete removal of all breast tissue from the area. However, the skin and underlying tissue, such as the nipple, lymph nodes, and pectoral muscles, are left intact. A **radical** mastectomy is similar to a simple complete mastectomy, but it also includes the removal of additional structures, such as the nipple, axillary or mammary lymph nodes, and pectoral muscle tissue.

These are typically used for the treatment or prevention of breast cancer. If the removal is performed for a reduction or to treat gynecomastia, different codes will be used. In addition, codes used in this section are used for single breasts. If the procedure involves both breasts, use modifier 50 in addition to the code.

Musculoskeletal System

MUSCULOSKELETAL SYSTEM

The musculoskeletal system is made up of two interlinked systems: the **muscular system,** which consists of the body's muscles; and the **skeletal system,** which consists of the body's bones. **Muscle** is soft tissue made up of protein filaments that can contract and relax when triggered by nerve impulses. Although there are three types of muscle in the human body, this section will focus on

skeletal muscles, or muscles attached to the skeleton. **Bones,** meanwhile, are dense and hard tissue made up of specialized cells in a calcium matrix. The skeleton can be divided into two major regions: the **axial** skeleton, which includes the skull, spine, rib cage, and sternum; and the **appendicular** skeleton, which includes the limbs, hands, feet, hips, and shoulders. This section also includes procedures involving **joints,** or places where bones meet and are linked together via connective tissue.

Many of the musculoskeletal system's major functions focus on the body's movement, posture, and shape. The body's skeleton provides a sturdy framework for the rest of the body's systems, as well as protecting vital organs from damage. Meanwhile, the body's muscles allow the body to move and balance, as well as define its shape and retain body heat.

PROCEDURES

Procedures involving the musculoskeletal system are covered by codes **20100** through **29999**, which are divided into related headings and subheadings throughout the section. Most of the headings are focused on a single anatomical location (e.g., head, hands, pelvis, and hips, etc.), and they will often contain similar procedures.

Procedures in this section include the following:

- Incisions and drainage of abscesses
- Excision of tumors or tissue, including **fasciotomy** (the cutting of connective tissue)
- **Radical resection**, or extensive removal of a tumor with significant margins of normal tissue
- Introduction of drugs or substances into joints
- Repair and reconstruction procedures, including prosthetics
- Treatment of fractures and dislocations
- **Manipulation**, or manual, physical movement of the body for treatment
- **Arthrodesis**, or surgical immobilization of a bone or joint
- **Amputation**, or surgical removal of part or all of a limb or extremity
- Applications of casts and other immobilizing devices
- **Arthroscopic** procedures, in which a thin, flexible scope enters a joint space for surgery or investigation.

OPEN, CLOSED, AND PERCUTANEOUS TREATMENT OF FRACTURES

CPT uses specific terms when discussing procedures treating fractures. **Closed treatment** is when a fracture is treated without surgically opening the location. Typically, this involves either manipulation or traction of the site. **Open treatment** is when the fractured bone is either surgically exposed for visualization or treatment, or when an area near the fracture is opened to insert a fixation device across the site. **Percutaneous treatment**, or **percutaneous skeletal fixation**, is when the fracture is neither open nor closed. Instead, fixation devices (such as pins) are inserted through the skin, typically while using X-ray imaging guidance. This terminology has no bearing on the type of fracture, merely on the treatment type.

TRAUMATIC WOUNDS

Traumatic wounds, meaning wounds resulting from penetrative trauma such as stabs and gunshots, are covered by codes **20100** through **20103**. These codes include the necessary processes involving exploration of the wound, enlargement of the wound opening, dissection to determine penetration, debridement and foreign body removal, and repair of minor subcutaneous and muscular blood vessels that do not require additional dedicated treatment.

However, if repairs are done using a thoracotomy or laparotomy, then those codes are reported instead. In addition, if the wound or wounds do not require exploration or enlargement, report the wound repair codes used in the integumentary system instead.

TRIGGER POINTS

A trigger point is a persistent and often painful knot of muscle, typically located along the back, neck, shoulders, or spine, that does not relax along with the rest of the muscle. Trigger points often accompany certain conditions such as an injury; fibromyalgia; or chronic neck, jaw, or lower back pain. When a trigger point is treated, a muscle-relaxing agent such as lidocaine or a corticosteroid is injected into the site, causing it to relax and dissipate.

When coding trigger point injections and similar procedures, it is important to note how many **muscles** are being treated, not the number of actual injections. For example, if 6 injections are performed on one muscle, and 4 injections are performed on another, then the code selection would be based on the two muscle sites, not the 10 injections. Additional codes will be required if imaging guidance is used during the treatment.

EXTERNAL FIXATION DEVICES

External fixation devices are used to correct and stabilize fractures or other bone defects. External fixation devices are attached to the bone through the skin via nails or pins, and they are bound to a metal frame that rests against or around the skin. Most such devices fall into three types:

- A **halo**, which attaches to the skull and is used typically for thin skull osteology
- A **uniplane external fixation system**, which is attached to a single bone or surface
- A **multiplane external fixation system**, which is attached to multiple bones or surfaces.

The type of device used varies depending on the severity, type, and location of the defect or fracture, and the procedure is usually done with anesthesia.

IMMOBILIZING DEVICES

Various immobilizing devices are used when treating fractures and dislocations in order to prevent further damage and to promote healing. CPT covers three different types of immobilization devices:

- **Casts**, protective shells made up of plastic, plaster, or fiberglass designed to protect the damaged location
- **Splints**, a length of hard material placed along a limb and then secured with bandages
- **Strapping**, overlapping strips of adhesive tape or bandages wrapped around the area.

When coding the use of immobilizing devices such as these, the initial cast used during part of a treatment is not coded. If it is performed afterward, or if it is separate from a treatment, then it should be coded. In addition, If the cast application or strapping is provided as the only initial care, then code **99070** should be used in addition to the relevant evaluation and management (E/M) code.

ENDOSCOPIC AND ARTHROSCOPIC PROCEDURES

Endoscopic procedures involve the use of a slender, flexible tube equipped with a light source, camera, and other tools (referred to as an **endoscope**) into a space inside the body. Endoscopic procedures are used for diagnostic or surgical purposes and are considered minimally invasive. Any surgical endoscopic procedure will, by necessity, include the services used in a diagnostic endoscopy; if there is a surgery involved, do not code a diagnostic endoscopy as well unless it is a completely separate service.

Arthroscopic procedures are a subset of endoscopies in which a scope is inserted into a joint for treatment and diagnosis. Arthroscopies can be performed on every major joint in the body, and they are listed in almost all sections of the musculoskeletal system. If an arthroscopy is performed with an **arthrotomy,** or surgical exploration, add modifier 51 to the arthroscopy code.

HEAD

Procedures involving the head (not including the skull) typically cover a few key anatomical sites. Common procedure sites on the head include the following:

- The **maxilla**, which forms the roof of the mouth and part of the eye sockets and nasal cavity
- The **mandibular rami,** the portion of the jawbone that curves upward behind the teeth
- The **temporomandibular joint**, the joint where the jawbone connects to the rest of the skull
- The **orbitals,** or the sections of bone that form the eye sockets
- The **scalp,** or the soft tissue on top of the head
- The **face,** which is typically involved in repair and reconstruction.

CODING FOR EXCISION OF NECK AND THORAX

When coding excision procedures on the soft tissue of the neck and the thorax, there are several factors to take into account:

First, check the **location** of the procedure, whether it is in the neck or the **chest wall,** which is made up of the ribs and sternum. Excision codes for the neck and the chest wall have different factors that must be taken into account.

For neck excision codes, check the **size** of the tumor being removed, which should be listed in centimeters (cm). In addition, check the **depth** of the tumor, whether it is subcutaneous or **subfascial** (below the muscle).

For chest wall excision codes, check the **subject** of the removal, such as a tumor or an actual rib. In addition, check if a **lymphadenectomy,** or a dissection of the lymph nodes, is being performed in addition to the removal.

CODING OF EXCISION OF BACK AND FLANK

Many of the codes dealing with the back and flank involve excision of soft tissue. Like most codes of similar procedures, there are a few key factors that must be accounted for in the procedure notes.

First, take the **depth** of the procedure into account, whether it is subcutaneous or subfascial. Afterward, check the **size** of the tumor being excised; CPT uses separate codes depending on if the mass is smaller than 5 cm or if it is 5 cm and larger.

When coding lesions that are cutaneous in origin (i.e., originating from the skin) and located on the back and flank, use codes located in the "Integumentary" section of CPT instead of codes in this section.

SPINE

The **spinal column** comprises a stack of 33 bones, called **vertebrae**, that run from the skull to the tailbone. The spinal column is divided into four areas depending on the location. Starting from the skull, there is the **cervical vertebrae** (C1 through C7) that support the head and form the neck, the **thoracic vertebrae** (T1 through T12) that connect to the ribs and form the upper back, the **lumbar vertebrae** (L1 through L5) that form the lower back, and the **sacrum** (S1 through S5) that are fused together and connect to the pelvic bones to form the hips and the **coccyx**, or tailbone, which is actually another 4 bones fused together.

Each **vertebra** shares several key features. Starting from the anterior portion is the large **vertebral body**, a thick piece of bone that forms most of the spine's mass and supports the pads of connective tissue known as **intervertebral discs**. Moving toward the posterior are the **pedicles**, which jut out from the body and link to the wing-like **transverse processes**. The transverse processes link into the **laminae,** which finally connect to the wedge-shaped **spinous processes**, which run along the posterior portion of the vertebrae. These arch-shaped protrusions help form the **spinal canal**, which the **spinal cord** runs through.

SPINAL ARTHRODESIS PROCEDURES

Spinal arthrodesis is the surgical fusion of two or more vertebrae, typically using grafted bone, in order to immobilize or stabilize vertebrae. Such procedures often include preparation procedures, a **discectomy** (the removal of the intervertebral disc), an **osteophytectomy** (the removal of any bone deposits or spurs), and possibly imaging guidance.

When coding these procedures, there are several key factors to take into account:

- First, confirm the **approach technique.** These procedures are divided up by how the spine is approached, such as through the back of the mouth or through the side of the neck.
- Next, confirm the **area of the spinal column** that is being immobilized. Depending on the approach, there may be a limited selection. An anterior transoral approach, for example, will only have the cervical vertebrae available to select from.
- After that, make note of the **number of interspaces** being immobilized. The **interspaces** are the spaces between vertebral bodies, so make sure not to confuse them with the vertebrae themselves. For example, the C2 to C3 vertebrae is one interspace.

SPINAL INSTRUMENTATION

Spinal instrumentation is the term used for prosthetic devices designed to support or stabilize damaged vertebrae and related structures. Spinal instrumentation includes the following devices:

- **Non-segmental spinal instrumentation**, typically a rod that is connected at either end to the spine
- **Segmental spinal instrumentation**, similar to non-segmental spinal instrumentation but connected to additional bony attachments
- **Intervertebral biomechanical device**, a synthetic cage or mesh attached to the vertebral body
- **Arthroplasty,** a synthetic intervertebral disc.

Instrumentation may or may not include spinal fusion, and it may span multiple vertebrae. Make note of which codes may or may not be used in conjunction with the codes used to report these procedures.

CODING FOR EXCISION OF ABDOMEN

Most procedures involving the abdomen focus on excision of tumors and similar masses located in or on the **abdominal wall**, the band of muscular and connective tissue that encompasses the abdomen and the organs contained within. When coding these procedures, check the **depth**, subcutaneous or subfascial, because different depths require different codes. In addition, when coding these excision codes, check the **size** of the tumor being removed, which should be listed in centimeters (cm). Multiple tumors will require additional codes because each code is meant for a single tumor.

If the lesions have a **cutaneous origin**, meaning they originate in the skin and not the actual abdominal tissue, then you will need to use codes from the Integumentary section of CPT.

CODING SHOULDER PROCEDURES

The shoulder is a complex system of joints formed at the intersection of three bones: the humerus, the scapula, and the clavicle. Together, these three bones form the two joints of the shoulder: the **glenohumeral joint**, which is formed where the rounded head of the humerus slots into the concave portion of the scapula; and the **acromioclavicular joint**, which is where the highest point of the scapula meets the clavicle. The shoulder section also covers the various muscles and tendons that make up what is referred to as the **rotator cuff**, which holds the head of the humerus in place and allows the arm to be rotated above the head.

CODING PROCEDURES OF ARM AND ELBOW

The **humerus** is the long bone that forms the upper part of the arm, connecting the shoulder to the forearm. Codes relating to the humerus and elbow covers the **shaft** (the long central portion) and the **distal** (furthest from the center of the body) end of the humerus. The humerus, alongside the proximal ends of the **radius** (the thinner forearm bone) and the **ulna** (the thicker, longer forearm bone) form the **elbow joint.** This section also covers procedures involving the **olecranon process**, which is the thick, proximal head of the ulna that forms the "bump" on the elbow; as well as the **lateral and medial epicondyles**, which are the rounded protrusions of the humerus.

CODING PROCEDURES OF ARM AND WRIST

Codes in this section refer to the shafts and distal ends of the **radius** (the thinner forearm bone) and the **ulna** (the thicker, longer forearm bone). These two bones form the forearm, which is then linked to the **wrist**. The wrist is a complex joint, made up of eight **carpal bones** and the associated connective tissue, which bridges the space between the forearm and the rest of the hand. Although there are several carpal bones, several procedures focus on the **scaphoid** and **lunate** bones, particularly when it comes to fractures. This is because those two bones are the closest to the forearm and are more likely to be damaged or fractured.

CODING PROCEDURES OF HAND AND FINGERS

Procedures listed in this section cover the structures of the hand. Working from the proximal end of the hand at the wrist, there are the **metacarpals**, a set of five bones that link to the wrist and form the basis for the fingers. From the metacarpals, we move into the **phalanges**, which form the actual fingers. There are 14 phalanges in total: three for each finger and two for the thumb. The phalanges are divided into the **proximal**, **middle**, and **distal phalanges**, the last of which carries the fingernail.

In terms of soft tissues, there are various muscles and tendons that allow the fingers to move and grip; and various joints, such as the **metacarpophalangeal** (metacarpal bones to phalanges) and **interphalangeal** (between the phalanges) joints.

CODING PROCEDURES OF PELVIS AND HIP

Procedures listed in this section cover the **pelvis**, the lowest part of the trunk. Similar to the shoulders, the pelvis is made up of multiple interlocking bones. Three bones form the ring-like structure of the pelvis, starting posteriorly with the **sacrum**, which links with the **coccyx** (tailbone) and connects to the spinal column. On either side of the sacrum are the **hip bones**, the large curved bones made up of three portions: the **ilium** (the wing-like crest), the **ischium** (the lower curved portion), and the **pubis** (the anterior curved portion that connects the hip bones together). These bones are important for supporting the body's weight and protecting the various organs of the lower body.

The pelvis is also the site of the **hip joint**, which is the ball-and-socket joint formed by the bowl-shaped socket in the hip bones called the **acetabulum**; and the rounded head of the femur. Other major joints covered by procedures in this section include the **sacroiliac**, the joint between the sacrum and the ilium of the hip bone; and the **symphysis pubis**, the joint between the pubis portion of the hip bones.

LEG

CODING PROCEDURES OF THIGH AND KNEE

The section covering the region of the upper leg commonly called the **thigh** is taken up by the **femur**, the long, thick bone that connects proximally to the pelvis and distally to the tibia and the lower leg. The femur is the longest bone of the body and consists of the **shaft**, or the long central piece; and the two rounded **epiphyses**, or extremities.

This section also includes the **knee**, a major hinge joint that is formed at the connection between the femur and the bones of the lower leg, particularly the tibia. The knee also includes the **patella**, the shield-like bone that forms the kneecap. Several codes also deal with the major joints of the knee, including the **tibiofemoral joint**, located between the femur and the tibia; the **patellofemoral joint**, located between the femur and the patella; and also the **meniscus**, or the jelly-like pad of connective tissue within the knee proper.

CODING PROCEDURES OF LOWER LEG AND ANKLE

The lower portion of the leg consists of two bones: the **tibia,** the thicker anterior medial bone that forms the **shin**; and the **fibula**, the thinner posterior lateral bone. These two bones function in a similar fashion to the radius and ulna, but they connect the knee to the ankle.

The **ankle** joint links the bones of the lower leg to the bones of the foot, specifically the **talus**. The ankle is made up of the **talocrural joint** between the talus and the tibia and fibula, the **subtalar joint** between the talus and the calcaneus, and the **inferior tibiofibular joint** between the tibia and the fibula at the lower portion. In addition to these major joints, several codes address procedures involving the **Achilles tendon,** the major tendon that runs along the back of the leg and the foot.

CODING PROCEDURES OF THE FEET AND TOES

The feet and toes are the most **inferior** (anatomically lowest) portion of the body. The feet and toes are similar in structure to the hand and wrist and are capable of similar movement. Moving from the proximal portion of the foot forward, there are the seven **tarsal** bones, including the **talus**; the **calcaneus**; the medial, intermediate and lateral **cuneiforms**; the **cuboid**; and the **navicular.** These bones help to form and connect the ankle joint to the rest of the foot, with the calcaneus forming the heel of the foot.

Proceeding along are the five **metatarsals**, which function similar to the metacarpals of the hand and connect the toes to the rest of the foot. Much like the hand, the foot terminates into 14 **phalanges**: two in the big toe and three in each other toe. Much like procedures of the hand, procedures of the foot cover treatment of several joints, such as the **metatarsophalangeal joint**, located between the metatarsals and the phalanges; and also soft tissue such as the **plantar fascia**, the connective tissue for the muscles on the bottom of the foot.

Respiratory System

ANATOMICAL STRUCTURES AND PROCEDURES

The respiratory system consists of the organs that provide oxygen to the rest of the body via breathing. Important structures involved in this section include the following:

- The **nose** and its associated structures, such as the **sinuses**
- The **larynx**, or voice box
- The **trachea**, the main tube that leads to the lungs and the **bronchi** that branch off of it
- The **lungs**, in which oxygen and carbon dioxide are exchanged and the blood is oxygenated; and the **pleura**, the membrane surrounding the lungs.

This section in CPT covers codes **30000** through **32999**, which include the following types of procedures:

- Incision, excision, introduction, repair, and destruction of tissues of the nose, larynx, trachea, bronchi, and lungs
- Endoscopies of the sinuses, larynx, trachea, bronchi, and lungs
- Video-assisted thoracic surgery of the lungs
- Lung transplants
- Therapeutic treatments of the lung, such as stereotactic radiation therapy and surgical collapse therapy.

VIDEO-ASSISTED THORACIC SURGERY AND RELATED PROCEDURES

Video-assisted thoracic surgery is a type of endoscopic surgery used for correcting issues of the **thorax** (chest). When a video-assisted thoracic surgery is performed, a flexible tube with a mounted light and camera, called an **endoscope**, is inserted through the thoracic cavity in order to directly inspect the lungs and allow surgical tools access without performing a more invasive procedure. Endoscopic procedures involving the thorax (especially the lungs) are also referred to as **thoracoscopies**.

A video-assisted thoracic surgery, particularly in this section, is performed for a variety of reasons, including the following:

- Biopsies of lung tissue and pleura
- Surgical excision of lesions on the lungs and pleura
- Removal or resection of lung, pleura, or lymph tissue
- Removal of excess fluid or air from the pleural area.

Cardiovascular System

ANATOMICAL STRUCTURES AND PROCEDURES

The cardiovascular system consists of the organs and systems that circulate blood, fluid, nutrients, and other substances throughout the body. It also removes waste products for disposal. Structures involved in this section include the following:

- The **heart**, the muscular pump that drives the system
- The **blood vessels**, which are divided into **arteries** that take blood away from the heart and **veins** that carry blood to the heart

- The **mediastinum**, the area around the trachea, esophagus, and the major blood vessels
- The **diaphragm**, the muscular wall that assists in breathing.

The cardiovascular system is covered by codes **33016** through **37799**, including the following procedures:

- Treatment and repair of conditions involving the heart and **pericardium** (heart membrane)
- Implanting devices, including defibrillators, monitors, and prosthetics
- Heart transplants
- Blood vessel repair and reconstruction
- Treatment of **aneurysms** (enlargements of artery wall) and **thromboses** (blood clots inside a blood vessel)
- Blood vessel grafting and transposition
- Preparation for and execution of **hemodialysis** (artificial filtering of waste from the blood).

PACEMAKER AND DEFIBRILLATOR PLACEMENT

Pacemakers, which help control abnormal heart rhythms; and **defibrillators**, which restore the heartbeat with an electrical shock, are common implants meant to treat heart conditions. When coding for these procedures, there are several factors that can influence the code required, including the following:

- The type of device (temporary pacemaker, implanted pacemaker, implanted defibrillator, etc.)
- Whether it is a new or replacement device (such as an upgrade from an older device) or the removal of a device
- The number of leads on the device (single, dual, or multiple leads)
- The method of insertion, such as via a thoracotomy or transcatheter.

Codes in this section also cover the repositioning of existing devices as well. Unless otherwise noted, the codes should also indicate the surgical procedures needed to insert or remove the device.

CABG

A coronary artery bypass graft (CABG) is a procedure in which blood vessels from other portions of the body are grafted to the heart and major vessels (the **aorta** and the **vena cava**) to allow for blood flow to reach tissues of the heart, typically due to poor or obstructed flow in the existing vessels.

There are two factors that must be considered when coding for a CABG. The first is the **type of graft** that is being used because that is what forms the initial categorization: **venous grafting** (in which veins are used), **arterial grafting** (in which arteries are used), or **combined arterial-venous grafting** (in which both types of tissue are used). When coding a combined grafting, the codes in the "Arterial Grafting" section (codes **33533** through **33548**) are used as the primary codes because the codes in the "Combined" section (**33517** through **33530**) are add-on codes. In addition, consider the **number of grafts**, which will determine the code used.

BYPASS GRAFTS OF BLOOD VESSELS

Bypass grafts are used to reroute blood around obstructions in a blood vessel. Typically, this is done by taking a portion of a blood vessel from another part of the body and transplanting it to the affected site, allowing blood flow to bypass the obstruction.

Much like when coding CABGs, there are certain factors that must be accounted for when coding bypass grafts. To begin with, check the **type of graft** being used. This includes a venous graft, an **in-situ vein** (rerouting through an existing vein), an arterial graft, or a **composite graft** (made of multiple different segments linked together). The other major factor is the **sites being linked**, such as a carotid-vertebral bypass, which determines the primary code. This section also includes add-on codes for the harvest of certain vessels for grafting procedures.

VENOUS AND ARTERIAL ORDERS

When coding certain cardiovascular procedures, such as **angiographies** (inspections of a blood vessel via a catheter), there will be mentions of "orders" of veins or arteries. **Orders** are a method of categorizing particular arteries or veins depending on their position in a grouping, known as a **vascular family.**

The best way to describe orders is to think of them like off-ramps of a highway. Each order is one "turnoff" away from the respective major vessels, the **aorta** and the **vena cava.** Thus, the **first order** is a branch off the major vessel, the **second order** is a branch off the first order, and so on. When coding a procedure involving orders, check what order the mentioned artery or vein is in the procedure description.

Refer to **Appendix L** in the CPT codebook for a map of vascular families and the various orders.

Hemic and Lymphatic

ANATOMICAL STRUCTURES AND PROCEDURES

The hemic and lymphatic system consists of the organs and tissues that help filter, maintain, and protect the body's blood supply. Procedures coded in this section include the following anatomical structures:

- The **spleen**, which filters the blood and removes dead or diseased cells
- **Bone marrow**, the spongy tissue inside bones that produces new blood cells
- **Stem cells**, undifferentiated cells used for repairing and building tissue
- The **lymph nodes**, nodules of tissue that filter **lymph fluid** and contain white blood cells
- The **lymph channels**, which circulate lymph fluid throughout the body.

Procedures involving the hemic and lymphatic systems are covered by codes **38100** through **38999** and include the following:

- Excision, repair, and laparoscopy of the spleen
- Procedures involving bone marrow or stem cells
- Transplant procedures
- Incision, excision, removal, and introduction of lymph nodes and related tissues.

Mediastinum and Diaphragm

ANATOMICAL STRUCTURES AND PROCEDURES

This section covers two separate anatomical structures: the mediastinum and the diaphragm. The **mediastinum** is the term used for the compartment that makes up the **thoracic cavity** and contains the heart and its vessels; esophagus; trachea; and all associated nerves, muscles, and lymph nodes. The mediastinum is bordered on the sides by the lungs and at the bottom by the diaphragm. The **diaphragm** is a sheet of skeletal muscle that stretches across the bottom of the thoracic cavity like a floor. The diaphragm not only separates the thoracic cavity, but it also contracts and expands to draw air into the lungs.

Procedures involving the mediastinum and the diaphragm are covered by codes **39000** through **39599** and include the following:

- Incision, excision, and endoscopy of the mediastinum
- Repair of the diaphragm.

Digestive System

ANATOMICAL STRUCTURES

The digestive system consists of a series of interlinked organs and associated systems that intake and digest nutrients, breaking them down to a form usable by the body, and then excrete any remaining waste matter. Digestion begins when nutrients are taken in to the mouth, past the lips, and are chewed before being swallowed. The mouth contains the **tongue, dentoalveolar structures** such as the teeth, the **palate** that forms the roof of the mouth and the dangling **uvula**, as well as **salivary glands and ducts.** Proceeding down from the mouth, food passes through the **pharynx**, down the **esophagus**, and into the **stomach**. It then passes through the stomach to the **duodenum**, as various enzymes from the **liver, gallbladder**, and **pancreas** are added to the mix. Food then passes through the rest of the **small intestine** (the **jejunum** and the **ileum**) before passing over the **appendix** and into the **large intestine**—made up of the **ascending, transverse,** and **sigmoid colons**—before waste is stored in the **rectum** and expelled through the **anus.**

PROCEDURES

Procedures involving the digestive system are covered by CPT codes **40490** through **49999**, which are divided into the related headings and subheadings throughout the section. Procedure codes will be grouped based on the anatomical location or system. Procedures in this section include the following:

- Incision, excision, and repair of various bodily structures
- Endoscopic investigation of the esophagus, intestines, colon, anus, and **biliary tract** (the connection between the liver, gallbladder, and intestine)
- **Laparoscopic** (endoscopy of the abdomen) procedures of the esophagus, stomach, intestines, appendix, colon, liver, biliary tract, and abdomen
- **Bariatric surgery** for purposes of weight loss
- Transplant surgery of the liver and pancreas
- Surgical repair of hernias.

LIPS

ANATOMICAL PURPOSE

The lips are the most external portion of the digestive system, and they serve as the primary opening for nutrient intake. The lips meet with the rest of the skin of the face at a point referred to as the **vermilion border**, and they consist of two fleshy protrusions controlled by facial muscles and containing nerves and blood vessels. In addition to allowing food intake and protecting the oral cavity and teeth from the outside environment, the lips assist in forming various speech sounds and facial expressions and serve as a tactile organ and as an additional erogenous zone due to their sensitivity.

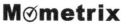

CHEILOPLASTY PROCEDURES

Cheiloplasty procedures refer to surgical procedures involving the repair and restoration of the lips. In CPT, cheiloplasty codes cover plastic surgery of the lips and the surgical correction of congenital **cleft lip**, a deformity that creates a split in the upper lip. When coding these procedures, note the type and purpose of the repair as well as the number of stages (if any) included in the procedure.

These codes are only for repairing the actual lip tissue and fixing cleft lips. Other reconstructive procedures will use codes from the integumentary system and are noted under the codes in this section.

MOUTH

ANATOMICAL STRUCTURES

The mouth is divided into two sections: the vestibule of the mouth and the oral cavity. The **vestibule of the mouth** is made up of all the parts outside of the dentoalveolar structures: the inner tissue of the cheeks and lips, the mucosal and submucosal portions thereof, and the space between them and the teeth. The **oral cavity** itself contains the teeth; gums; tongue; and the **floor of the mouth**, which is the fleshy tissue underneath the tongue. Because much of the mouth's interior consists of soft tissue, most of the codes involving it revolve around removing lesions and masses and repairing damage from trauma or defects.

DENTOALVEOLAR STRUCTURES

Dentoalveolar structures refer to the structures including and surrounding the teeth, **gingiva** (the gums), and associated structures such as the **alveolar process** (the bony sockets that hold the teeth). These structures are designed to chew and tear through food, allowing it to be digested easily and increase its exposure to saliva.

Most of the codes in this section cover the excision of lesions or foreign bodies from the soft tissue and repair of gum tissues and both soft and bony portions of the alveolar process. These codes do not involve actual dental procedures, only surgical ones; dental procedures are described in a completely separate text.

PALATE AND UVULA

The **palate** is the bone and tissue that form the roof of the mouth, separating the oral cavity from the nasal cavity above it. The palate consists of a layer of mucosal and soft tissue (the **soft palate**) that covers the harder bone (the **hard palate**) just above. Codes involving the palate typically refer to destruction of soft tissue and masses and the repair of a **cleft palate**, which is an opening (typically congenital) in the palate.

The **uvula** (also known as the palatine uvula) is the downward-hanging flap of tissue located near the back of the mouth. In addition to helping produce saliva, the uvula helps to close off and prevent food from entering the **nasopharynx**, the opening that leads to the nasal cavity. Codes involving the uvula involve excisions of lesions and the uvula itself.

SALIVARY GLANDS AND DUCTS

The **salivary glands** are specialized glands located in the mouth that produce **saliva**, a fluid that helps lubricate food while it is chewed. In addition to hundreds of minor salivary glands, the mouth has three pairs of major salivary glands: the **parotid** (on the side of the face behind the jaw), **submandibular** (below the jaw), and the **sublingual** (below the tongue) glands. Saliva is carried from the glands to the mouth via **salivary ducts**.

This section deals mostly with soft tissue, which is reflected by the procedures listed. Most of the codes in this section involve the treatment of abscesses; the excision of cysts, tumors, and glands; and the repair of salivary ducts.

PHARYNX, ADENOIDS, AND TONSILS

The **pharynx** is the chamber located directly behind the mouth, which connects the mouth and nasal cavities to the esophagus and larynx. In addition to serving as a point of connection, the pharynx helps with speech.

The **adenoids** and **tonsils** are part of the lymphatic system located in the pharynx. The adenoids are located behind and on either side of the uvula on the roof of the pharynx, whereas the tonsils are located at the rear of the pharynx inside the lateral walls and behind the tongue. The adenoids and tonsils help to capture and eliminate inhaled and ingested bacteria.

TONSILLECTOMY AND ADENOIDECTOMY PROCEDURES

Tonsillectomies and adenoidectomies are the surgical removal of the tonsils and adenoids, typically due to chronic infection or obstruction of the esophagus or larynx. Although this is typically done on younger patients, it can be performed on adults as well. When coding these procedures, there are several factors that must be taken into account when selecting the correct code. First, check **what is being removed**, whether it is the tonsils, the adenoids, or both. Additionally, check the **patient's age**. Different codes are used when the patient is age 12 and older. In addition, check if this is a **radical resection**, which involves the removal of the tonsils and additional surrounding tissues.

ESOPHAGUS

The esophagus is a tube of fibrous and muscular tissue that connects the pharynx to the stomach. The esophagus runs down behind the heart through the mediastinum and the diaphragm before connecting to the uppermost part of the stomach. Food is passed down the esophagus via muscular contractions, and a pair of **sphincters** (muscular gates) prevent food and stomach contents from flowing back toward the mouth.

Procedures involving the esophagus include excision of masses and tissue, endoscopic procedures of the esophagus and passing through it, laparoscopic procedures of the esophagus and the upper portion of the stomach, repair procedures (including the insertion of prosthetics), and manipulation of the esophageal structure.

ENDOSCOPIC PROCEDURES

The esophagus is involved in a variety of endoscopic procedures due to its easy access via the mouth and its connection to the stomach. The procedures listed in this section are divided into three types: **esophagoscopy**, or endoscopic inspection and procedures of the esophagus itself; **esophagogastroduodenoscopy**, which is an endoscopic procedure involving the gastrointestinal tract from the esophagus, through the stomach, and into the duodenum; and **endoscopic retrograde cholangiopancreatography**, a combination of endoscopy and fluoroscopy used to diagnose and treat issues of the pancreatic and biliary ducts.

There are several important factors to take into consideration when coding these procedures. For esophagoscopies, check the **point of entry** (oral, nasal, etc.), the **type of scope** (rigid or flexible), and **any additional procedures** (biopsy, removal of lesions, dilation, etc.). For **esophagogastroduodenoscopies**, check which **procedures** are performed (e.g., removal of foreign bodies, injections, etc.). Finally, for **endoscopic retrograde cholangiopancreatography**, check which **procedures** are being performed. In addition, many of the procedure codes come with a list of even more codes that are not to be reported alongside them (e.g., do not report 43263 in conjunction with 43260).

STOMACH
ANATOMY AND PROCEDURES

The stomach is a hollow, flexible, muscular organ that rests in the left upper quadrant of the abdomen and connects to the esophagus and the small intestine. The stomach can be separated into four sections: the **cardia**, which connects to the esophagus; the **fundus**, or upper curved portion; the **body**, which makes up the central region of the stomach; and the **pylorus**, which connects to the small intestine at the duodenum. The stomach's purpose is to break down chewed food for digestion via the secretion of enzymes and acid.

Procedures involving the stomach include incisions into the stomach, surgical removal of tissues, laparoscopic procedures, **gastric intubation** (insertion of a tube into the stomach via the nose or mouth), **bariatric surgery** (surgery involving the stomach and portions of the small intestine), and the insertion or removal of implanted devices.

GASTRIC BYPASS PROCEDURES

Gastric bypass procedures are surgical procedures in which a large portion of the stomach is surgically bypassed, leaving a smaller pouch that is connected to the small intestine. This is typically done to treat morbid obesity and related conditions. Gastric bypass procedures are included in a variety of codes in this section, mostly for procedures meant to treat obesity. When coding these sorts of procedures, check if the procedure notes mention a **Roux-en-Y gastroenterostomy**. A Roux-en-Y procedure is a specific procedure in which the small intestine is divided and rearranged into a Y shape and connected to the stomach. Procedures that use the Roux-en-Y approach require different codes than standard bypass procedures.

INTESTINES
ANATOMY

The intestines are long, hollow muscular organs that aid digestion by extracting nutrients from digested food and by moving solid waste toward the rectum and anus for excretion. The intestines are made up of two distinct organs.

The first is the **small intestine**, which handles most of the absorption. The small intestine is divided into three distinct regions: the **duodenum**, which connects to the stomach; the **jejunum**, which makes up the upper portion; and the **ileum**, the bottom portion that connects to the large intestine.

The second is the **large intestine**, which helps extract water and salt and moves solid waste to the end of the digestive tract. The large intestine can be divided into six sections: the **cecum**, which connects the large intestine to the end of the small intestine; the **ascending colon**, which moves waste upward; the **transverse colon**, which goes across the upper part of the abdomen; the **descending colon**; and the **sigmoid colon**, which connects to the **rectum**.

COLECTOMY

A colectomy is a surgical procedure involving the removal of part or all of the large intestine for the purpose of treating diseases or ongoing issues. Colectomy procedures are surgical, and they can be done either openly or via a laparoscopic approach. There are several factors that must be accounted for when a colectomy procedure is coded. The first matter is whether the colectomy is done

surgically or via a laparoscope. Next, check whether the procedure is either **partial or total**, meaning whether part or all of the large intestine is removed. Finally, check what **other procedures** are included, such as a **colostomy** (connecting the colon to an opening in the body) or an **anastomosis** (connecting two parts of the colon together).

STOMAL ENDOSCOPY

A **colonoscopy through a stoma,** or stomal endoscopy, is when an endoscopic procedure enters the intestine through a **stoma,** an artificially created opening in the body. In this case, the stoma is typically a percutaneous opening from the colon to the outside of the body, or a **colostomy.** These procedures involve examination or treatment through the ileum and all the way to the cecum.

There are several factors to take into account when coding these procedures. In particular, attention should be paid to the **location being studied** (i.e., the ileum or the entire colon). Next, pay attention to what, if any, additional procedures are performed during the procedure.

Colonoscopies other than through a stoma can be found in the "Rectum" heading of CPT.

APPENDIX

The appendix is a small, tube-like organ that protrudes just below the cecum located in the lower right quadrant of the abdomen. The appendix functions as a reservoir for beneficial gut bacteria, and it serves as a part of the immune and lymphatic systems.

Procedures involving the appendix almost entirely revolve around its removal, typically related to appendicitis and similar conditions that, if left untreated, could cause significant danger to the patient when the appendix ruptures. Removal of the appendix can be performed surgically or laparoscopically. These codes are not reported if the appendix is removed as part of a different procedure unless its removal is relevant. If it is, use modifier 52 with the removal code.

RECTUM

The rectum is the short, straightened end of the large intestine that connects the sigmoid colon to the anus. The rectum's purpose is to act as a storage site for fecal material received from the colon before it is expelled through the anus. Because of its location and connection to the anus, the rectum is a common entry point for some procedures seeking to access the intestines. Procedures involving the rectum include the removal of tumors and masses, surgical removal of portions of rectal tissue, colonoscopies, laparoscopic procedures, repair of damaged tissues, and manipulation of the anus and impacted fecal material.

COLONOSCOPIES

Colonoscopies are endoscopic procedures in which the endoscope enters the large intestine via the rectum for diagnostic or treatment purposes. This section deals with three distinct types of colonoscopy procedures, which vary based on how far the endoscope travels through the large intestine. A **proctosigmoidoscopy** is when the scope only examines the rectum and part of the sigmoid colon. A **sigmoidoscopy** is when the scope examines the entire rectum and sigmoid colon and may include part of the descending colon. A **colonoscopy** is when the entire large intestine, from rectum to cecum, is examined and may include examination of the terminal ileum.

Colonoscopies can also include an examination through a stoma. Codes for this particular procedure can be found in the "Intestine" section, starting with code **44388**. When coding these procedures, note which procedures are performed, if any.

ANUS

The anus is the opening at the end of the digestive tract, completely opposite of the mouth. The purpose of the anus is to control the expulsion of **feces**, or solid waste products that are produced from the unwanted or unhealthy matter left over from digestion. The anus is the terminus of the large intestine and includes the **anal canal**, which is the open space between the **inner** and **outer anal sphincters**.

Procedures involving the anus include incisions for treatment of fistulas and perineal abscesses, excision of hemorrhoids, endoscopic procedures for tumor removal, repair of damage, and destruction of anal lesions.

HEMORRHOIDECTOMY

Procedures for the treatment of hemorrhoids, or swollen vascular structures in and around the anal canal, are covered in the "Anal" portion of the "Digestive" section. Treatment of this problem is typically done with a **hemorrhoidectomy**, or surgical removal of hemorrhoid tissue. When coding procedures involving the removal of hemorrhoids, pay attention to certain key factors in the procedure. First, check if the hemorrhoid being removed is **internal**, **external**, or **both**. If internal, check which **method** is being used, such as ligation or dearterialization. If external or both internal and external, check on the **number of groups** that are being removed.

LIVER

ANATOMY AND PROCEDURES

The liver is a large, four-lobed organ that is located in the right upper quadrant of the abdomen. As an **accessory organ** (an organ that assists, but isn't directly involved) of the digestive system, the liver helps to metabolize carbohydrates, proteins, amino acids, and lipids; it breaks down many waste products and toxic substances such as alcohol; and it produces **bile**, a yellowish fluid that helps emulsify consumed fat. The liver is connected to the gallbladder and small intestine via the **common hepatic duct.**

Procedures involving the liver include biopsies, excisions, surgical removal of portions of the liver, transplants, repair of cysts and bleeding, laparoscopic treatments, and ablation of tumors through various methods.

LIVER TRANSPLANT

Liver transplants are a type of **allograft**, a graft or transplant that originates from a donor of the same species. Because the liver's numerous functions cannot be replicated with a prosthetic, a liver transplant is used to treat major issues such as acute liver failure. Liver transplant procedures require the careful consideration of several factors when reading the procedural notes in order to select the proper code. The first and major factor is the **source** of the transplanted tissue. If the source is from a living donor, then the actual removal of tissue, or **hepatectomy**, must be taken to account, as well as which **segments** of the liver are removed. If the source is from a cadaver, then the **backbench work**, or surgical removal and preparation, must be coded.

BILIARY TRACT

ANATOMY AND PROCEDURES

The biliary tract (also called the **biliary system**) is a series of ducts and canals that connect the liver and gallbladder to the small intestine at the duodenum. The biliary tract is the path by which bile is transported from the liver into the small intestine. The **gallbladder** is included in this system because it is an accessory organ that stores bile when not in use. The biliary tract is made up of the **common hepatic duct**, into which the bile produced by the ducts and canals in the liver flows,

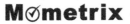

which then joins the **cystic duct** from the gallbladder to form the **common bile duct**, which joins with the pancreatic duct and enters the small intestine through the **ampulla of Vater.**

Procedures included in this section include the placement of implants and manipulation, endoscopic procedures, removal of the gallbladder, and repair of the biliary tract's structures.

EXCHANGE AND CONVERSION PROCEDURES INVOLVING BILIARY TRACT DRAINS AND STENTS

The "Biliary Tract" section covers the placement of catheters and stents for the purposes of treatment. Biliary drainage catheters are used to drain bile out of the body when a bile duct is damaged or blocked, usually on a temporary basis. However, providers may decide to switch from a drain to a more permanent stent, depending on the duct's condition or the treatment plan. **Stents**, meanwhile, are flexible metal tubing or mesh designed to hold a duct open to correct blockages or aid in drainage, and they are meant to be used long term. When coding these exchanges, check the chart located in the "Biliary Tract" subheading in this section. In addition, several codes have their own separate code sequences, listed under each description, that note which codes shouldn't be reported in conjunction with placement or removal codes.

PANCREAS

The pancreas is an abdominal organ located behind the stomach that plays an important role in the endocrine and digestive systems. In addition to producing a variety of important hormones for the body, the pancreas aids the digestive system by producing **pancreatic juice** that neutralizes stomach acid and helps to break down carbohydrates, protein, and fat. The pancreas is linked to the small intestine via the **pancreatic duct,** which links to the common bile duct before it enters the ampulla of Vater.

Procedures involving the pancreas include biopsies of pancreatic tissue, removal of tissue and the ampulla of Vater, injections for radiographic study, and repair of pancreatic structures and transplants.

ABDOMEN, PERITONEUM, AND OMENTUM

The **abdomen**, or abdominal cavity, is the large body cavity located just below the thorax (or chest) and above the pelvis. The abdomen is the area that contains a variety of important organs, including the stomach, liver, intestines, gallbladder, pancreas, spleen, and kidneys. The upper boundary of the abdomen is formed by the diaphragm, whereas its floor is made up of the pelvic inlet.

The abdomen is enclosed by the **abdominal wall**, a three-layered wall of muscle that protects the organs inside and helps to maintain the body's shape. Just past the abdominal wall is the **peritoneum**, a large serous membrane that lines the inside of the abdominal cavity. The peritoneum is divided into two layers: the **parietal peritoneum**, which attaches to the abdominal wall; and the **visceral peritoneum**, which cushions and supports the various abdominal organs and their blood, lymph, and nervous connections. The peritoneum also includes the **greater and lesser omenta**, which enclose nerves, blood, lymph vessels, and connective tissue for the transverse colon and the curve of the stomach and the space between the stomach and liver, respectively.

ABDOMINAL HERNIA REPAIR

Hernias are abnormal exits or protrusions of an organ or organ tissue, such as intestines or the colon, through the wall of the cavity that contains it. The most common hernias involve the abdominal area, including the **groin**, which is the area where the abdomen ends and the legs begin.

35

Hernias are typically repaired surgically, and they often include the insertion of prosthetic mesh to repair the opening.

There are several factors to keep in mind when coding hernia repair procedures. These include the **patient's age** (because some hernias occur in younger patients), the **type of hernia** based on its location (such as inguinal or umbilical), whether the hernia is **initial or recurrent** (first time versus previously repaired), if the hernia is **incarcerated** (trapped) or **strangulated** (the blood flow is cut off), and the **method of repair** (such as surgical or laparoscopic).

The use of surgical mesh is included in almost all of these repair codes, except for codes **49560** through **49566**. When using those codes, report the mesh separately.

Urinary System

ANATOMICAL STRUCTURES

The urinary system consists of a series of interlinked organs and vessels that eliminate fluid waste from the body in the form of **urine**. In doing so, the system helps to control the levels of electrolytes and metabolites in the body as well as regulating blood volume, pressure, and pH. The organs involved in this system are located in the abdomen and pelvis. Starting from the superior position, there are the **kidneys**, the bean-shaped organs that sit near the back of the abdominal cavity and filter the bloodstream. Wastes such as urea and uric acid then flow out of the kidneys through tubes of smooth muscle called **ureters**, which flow down into the **urinary bladder** located in the pelvic cavity. The bladder then stores urine until it is expelled through the **urethra**, another muscular tube that leads to the outside of the body.

PROCEDURES

Procedures involving the urinary system are covered by codes **50010** through **53899** and are divided by anatomical location within the system. Procedures included in this section include the following:

- Incision and excision of masses and lesions in the kidneys, ureter, bladder, and urethra
- Kidney transplants
- Introduction of substances and prosthetics into the system's structures
- Urodynamic procedures
- Repairing damaged tissue
- Laparoscopic procedures, including surgery
- Endoscopic procedures
- Transurethral surgical procedures
- Procedures involving the prostate, including resection or destruction of tissue
- Manipulation of the urethra for treatment purposes.

It should be noted that, other than procedures involving the prostate, the procedures are identical regardless of the gender of the patient.

CYSTOSCOPY

Endoscopic procedures involving the urinary system (typically including the bladder) are usually referred to as cystoscopies. This section also includes **urethroscopies**, which include the urethra; as well as **cystourethroscopies**, which include the urethra, bladder, and ureter. These procedures cover diagnostic and surgical procedures involving the endoscopy. As always, diagnostic procedures are included in procedures meant for treatment.

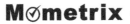

When coding these procedures, it's important to note the **type of procedure** being performed because each one covers different depths of the urinary system. In addition, take note of the **additional procedures** performed during the endoscopy, such as insertions of stents or treatment of intrarenal strictures. Also, record any parenthetical notes beneath the procedure descriptions because some codes are not reported in conjunction with other codes.

TRANSURETHRAL RESECTION OF PROSTATE

A transurethral resection of the prostate is a type of surgical procedure used to remove or eliminate prostate tissue that obstructs the urethra, preventing normal expelling of urine. Because this is a procedure involving the prostate, it will only be performed on biologically male patients. There are a few factors to consider when coding these particular procedures. The first factor is whether it is a **partial or total resection**, with total resection involving the complete removal of the prostate. The second factor when coding this type of procedure is whether this is the initial encounter for the procedure or if this is a recurrent procedure to treat residual or regrown tissue.

Similar codes in the same section, particularly **52647** through **52649,** include this procedure along with several others. Consider the notes listed in parentheses underneath the descriptions of each code.

Male Reproductive System

ANATOMICAL STRUCTURES

The male reproductive system is made up of the sexual organs possessed by biologically male individuals. These organs are located in the pelvic region, and they are designed to assist in reproduction by producing semen and as erogenous zones. Semen production begins in the **testes**, which are suspended in an external, fleshy sac called the **scrotum**. Semen flows into the **epididymis**, where it is stored until use. Semen then flows through the **vas deferens**, or deferent duct, up and around until it joins with the **ejaculatory duct**. In the ejaculatory duct, the semen is mixed with fluid produced by the **seminal vesicle** and the **prostate** before being expressed into and through the urethra. The male urethra passes through the **penis**, the tube-shaped external reproductive and sexual organ.

CIRCUMCISION

Circumcision is a type of excision procedure involving the surgical removal of the male **foreskin**. The foreskin is a double-layered fold of skin, muscle tissue, blood vessels, nerves, and mucous membrane that covers the penis and protects it from abrasion. Circumcision is typically performed at a very young age, often following birth, for cultural or religious reasons. In some cases, uncircumcised adults are circumcised due to medical necessity or during treatment for a related condition of the genitalia. Because of this, the **age of the patient** is a major factor when coding circumcision procedures: Most circumcision codes involve patients that are 28 days old or younger. In addition to age, the **method** of circumcision is also important. Note the method that is used and code appropriately.

PROSTATE REMOVAL

The prostate is a gland located around the urethra just before the penis that produces fluid and constricts the portion of the urethra leading to the bladder during ejaculation. Prostate removal procedures, or **prostatectomies**, are performed in the event that the prostate becomes cancerous. There are several factors to take into account when selecting the proper codes for these procedures. The first factor is the **approach**, which is how the prostate is accessed during the procedure. The next factor to consider is the **level of removal**: whether the procedure is subtotal

37

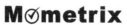

(partial) or radical (complete, including removal of additional tissue). Finally, make note of any **additional procedures**, such as lymph node biopsies, that are performed during the procedure. The procedure may automatically include certain other procedures, such as vasectomies, in the code. Included procedures should not be coded separately.

Female Reproductive System

ANATOMICAL STRUCTURES

The female reproductive system is made up of the sexual organs possessed by biologically female individuals. These organs are located in the pelvic region and assist in reproduction by producing eggs, carrying fertilized eggs to term, and also include erogenous zones. Starting from the organs involved in production, the system begins with the **ovaries**, which produce and store unfertilized eggs. These eggs are released from the ovaries and are captured by the **infundibulum**, the open, funnel-like portion of the **fallopian** (or uterine) **tubes.** The egg then moves down through the **ampulla** and into the fallopian tube proper before entering the **uterus**, the large, open organ where reproduction takes place. The uterus is linked to the **cervix** (the flexible, sphincter-like opening) by the **cervical canal.** Past the cervix lies the **vagina**, the tube-like opening that leads out of the body. The vagina then terminates at the external female sex organs, including the **vulva.**

EXCISION PROCEDURES OF VULVA

When coding excision procedures of the vulva, or **vulvectomies**, it is important to recognize the common terms used when describing the procedures. There are four particular terms used when describing the procedures, which are defined as the following:

- **Simple** vulvectomy procedures involve the removal of skin and superficial tissue and are the least intensive types of procedures.
- **Radical** vulvectomy procedures involve the removal of the skin, superficial tissue, and deeper subcutaneous tissue and are much more intensive and involved.
- **Partial** vulvectomy procedures involve the removal of less than 80 percent of the vulvar area.
- **Complete** vulvectomy procedures involve the removal of 80 percent or more of the vulvar area.

These codes are only for the actual removal procedures. Additional procedures, such as skin grafts or biopsies, will require additional codes.

HYSTERECTOMY

A hysterectomy is a surgical procedure that involves the removal of the uterus, typically for therapeutic or treatment-related reasons. As with most intensive surgical procedures, it is important to read the procedural notes and consider several factors when coding them. The first is the **approach** of the surgery: whether the procedure is performed via a **supracervical** (an incision above the cervix) or **vaginal** (through the vaginal canal) approach. Also, check if the procedure is surgical or laparoscopic: Laparoscopic hysterectomy procedures are found in the "Laparoscopic" section. Next, check what **other structures** are removed, such as the vagina or ovaries. For vaginal approaches, the removal of additional structures is labeled under separate codes.

MATERNITY AND DELIVERY

Most procedures involved in the "Maternity Care" section of CPT include **antepartum**, or prebirth, procedures and services. These procedures typically include prenatal history and examination, recording of the fetus's vital signs, routine urinalysis, and visits until the date of delivery. This section includes diagnostic and therapeutic **amniocentesis**, or extraction of amniotic fluid, as well as infusions and repair procedures.

The "Maternity Care" section also includes the treatment of **ectopic pregnancies**, which are when an otherwise viable fertilized egg implants outside of the uterus, such as on the ovary or inside the fallopian tube. These typically require surgical or laparoscopic intervention, and they often include relevant preparatory procedures.

DELIVERY

Procedures involving delivery, or the actual physical process of childbirth, are coded in multiple ways based on a number of factors. The first and most obvious one is the **method of delivery**. This covers traditional vaginal delivery, i.e., with no complications or intervention; as well as **Cesarean delivery**, which involves surgical intervention. Deliveries that occur after a previous Cesarean delivery are coded with different codes than a vaginal delivery.

In the case of uncomplicated maternity cases, delivery codes are bundled in along with antepartum and postpartum care. This applies to certain codes such as 59400.

ABORTION

Abortion is a term used for the predelivery termination of a pregnancy. Abortions can be caused artificially by a provider or can result from bodily functions, trauma, or diseases (which are commonly referred to as **miscarriages**). Abortions discussed in CPT include the following:

- **Incomplete abortion**, in which some of the products of conception remain inside the body
- **Missed abortion**, in which the products of conception remain inside the body
- **Septic abortion**, resulting from an infection of the uterus
- **Induced abortion**, in which the abortion is caused by medical intervention

When coding abortion procedures, check the type of abortion, the **method of treatment**, and (in some cases) the **trimester** and **additional procedures**. For a spontaneous abortion, check codes **99201** through **99233** for the appropriate procedure codes.

Endocrine System

ANATOMICAL STRUCTURES

The endocrine system is a series of glands and organs that create and maintain multiple chemical reactions and feedback loops within the body. This is done by producing the necessary hormones for the body, which in turn regulate physiological, developmental, and behavioral processes. Major organs that are considered part of the endocrine system include the following:

- Thyroid glands, located in the neck on either side of the trachea
- Parathyroid glands, smaller glands attached to the back of the thyroid
- Adrenal glands, located above the kidneys
- Pancreas
- Carotid body, near the fork of the carotid artery in the neck
- Ovaries (in females) and testes (in males).

Procedures involving the endocrine system are covered by codes **60000** through **60699.**

THYROIDECTOMY

A thyroidectomy is the surgical removal of part or all of the thyroid gland for the purposes of treatment or removal of diseased tissue. A related procedure is the **thyroid lobectomy**, which involves the removal of the thyroid from one side of the neck. When coding these types of procedures, there are a few important factors that must be taken into account. The first of these is the **amount of tissue** being removed. If only one lobe of the thyroid is removed, it's a **lobectomy**; if the entire thyroid is being removed either partially (**subtotal**) or completely (**total**), it is a thyroidectomy. Check which **additional procedures** are included, such as a contralateral subtotal lobectomy or dissection of the lymph nodes of the neck.

Nervous System

ANATOMICAL STRUCTURES

The nervous system is the complex, interlinked system of tissues and organs that transmits and receives the signals that control all bodily functions, both conscious and unconscious. The nervous system is divided into two parts: the **central nervous system** and the **peripheral nervous system.**

The central nervous system consists of the **brain,** the large mass of neural matter located inside the skull that controls the body; and the **spinal cord**, a long tubular structure that runs down along the vertebrae through the **spinal canal**, the open space behind the vertebral bodies. The central nervous system serves as the body's main control center and communication system. The peripheral nervous system is the term used for all of the other nerves that branch off of the spinal cord, which control the various muscles, organs, and other systems within the body.

PROCEDURES

Procedures involving the nervous system and its associated structures are covered by CPT codes **61000** through **64999** in the CPT handbook, which are divided into related headings and subheadings throughout the section based on anatomical relevance. Procedures in this section include the following:

- Injection, drainage, and aspiration procedures on the skull, spine, and nerves
- Surgery of the skull, base of the skull, and brain
- Surgical treatment of aneurysms and other vascular disease of the brain
- Implanting of neurostimulators and other devices
- Decompression of the spinal cord and other nerves
- Excision of spinal cord lesions
- Stereotactic radiosurgery of the brain and spinal cord
- Chemical destruction of nerves (aka **chemodenervation**)
- **Neurorrhaphy**, the surgical rejoining of split nerves
- Nerve grafts.

SKULL

CRANIAL PUNCTURE PROCEDURES

Holes are sometimes created in the skull in order to facilitate access to the tissues within or to treat issues inside the skull. The codes that cover these sorts of procedures are **61105** through **61253** in CPT, and they often include other procedures such as biopsies. There are several factors that must be taken into account when coding these procedures. First, and most importantly, the **type of tool** that is used to create the opening: a **twist drill** (a standard drilling tool), a **burr hole** (created using

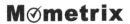

a surgical drill), or a **trephine** (a specialized manual tool). Following that, the next most important factor is the **procedure** involved with the creation of the hole, such as a biopsy or aspiration of a hematoma.

SURGICAL PROCEDURES INVOLVING BASE OF SKULL

Surgeries involving the base of the skull where the brain rests, also known as the **cranial fossa**, are extremely intensive and require multiple surgeons working together. In the CPT handbook, these procedures are divided into three specific categories that typically occur in sequence, one after another. The first is the **approach**, which is how the surgeons enter the location they're working in. These procedures are divided depending on the fossa in question: anterior, middle, or posterior. Next is the **definitive procedure**, which involves the surgical correction of the issue and primary closure. Last is the **repair/reconstruction**, in which the openings that were created are fixed and repaired via grafts or other procedures. If a single surgeon performs more than one procedure, add the modifier 51 to the secondary procedure or procedures.

MENINGES

The brain and spinal cord do not rest directly against the bones protecting them. The brain and the spinal cord are covered with a protective series of membranes referred to as the **meninges.** The meninges are made up of three layers: the **dura mater**, the outermost layer that rests against the bones of the skull and the vertebrae and contains the blood supply; the **arachnoid mater**, which is a thin connective layer that forms the boundary between the outer and inner layers of the meninges; and the **pia mater**, the thin and delicate membrane that attaches to the brain and spinal cord. The space between the pia mater and the arachnoid mater is referred to as the **subarachnoid space** and contains **cerebrospinal fluid (CSF)**, a colorless fluid that provides a cushioning effect.

BRAIN

ANATOMY

The brain is a highly complex organ, located inside the skull, that serves as the central point of the nervous system, effectively functioning as a biological computer in control of all of the body's other organs and systems. In CPT, the brain is divided into two **hemispheres** (left and right) and consists of six regions: the **frontal lobes** (the large and frontmost part of the brain), the **parietal lobes** (the middle of the brain), the **temporal lobes** (located to the sides and below the parietal lobes), the **occipital lobes** (located toward the rear of the skull), the **cerebellum** (the mass located just below the occipital lobes), and the **brain stem** (where the brain meets the spinal cord). The brain also contains a variety of other structures and glands, such as the **hypothalamus, thalamus, pituitary gland, pons**, and **medulla**, that help to regulate the body's various hormonal systems.

SURGICAL TREATMENT OF ANEURYSMS AND RELATED CONDITIONS

Issues involving the blood vessels of the brain typically require surgical intervention, which in CPT are covered by codes **61680** through **61711**. These codes cover the treatment of aneurysms, **arteriovenous malformation** (a tangle of connected arteries and veins), and other vascular diseases such as **fistulas** (abnormal connections between two spaces, such as blood vessels). There are several factors to take into account when coding these procedures. First, confirm the **issue being fixed**, such as a malformation or aneurysm. For malformations, check the **location** (supratentorial, infratentorial or dural) and whether it's **simple** or **complex.** For aneurysms, check the **approach** (e.g., intracranial, cervical, etc.) in order to select the correct code.

PROCEDURES INVOLVING CEREBROSPINAL FLUID (CSF) SHUNTS

A cerebrospinal fluid (CSF) shunt is a medical implant that is placed inside the body in order to relieve pressure on the brain caused by an excess of CSF. Procedures involving CSF shunts typically

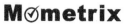

involve either the placement of a new shunt, the replacement or revision (such as for an obstructed valve) of an existing shunt, or the complete removal of the system without replacement. In addition to those general categories, it is important to take several factors into account when coding these procedures. When a shunt is being placed, confirm the **location of the shunt** and the **method** with which it is placed. In addition, pay attention to the parenthetical notes under the replacement and revision and complete removal procedure codes.

SPINE

SPINAL PUNCTURE PROCEDURES

Spinal puncture procedures use a needle or similar tool that is inserted into the spinal canal for treatment purposes, typically involving injections, drainage, or aspiration. Injections into the spine typically involve injections into the **spinal epidural space**, which is a layer between the dura mater and the actual bony portion of the spine. These procedures are often referred to as **epidurals**, and they can involve the injection of contrast agents, therapeutic drugs, or anesthetics. Aspiration of the spine, or a **spinal tap**, is the removal of CSF or other material from the spine, whereas drainage involves removal of excess CSF.

When coding these procedures, note the key terms used by CPT in describing the procedure. These terms cover the **method** (percutaneous, endoscopic, and open) and **method of visualization** (either **indirect** via imaging guidance or **direct** via eyesight or endoscope).

LAMINOTOMY AND LAMINECTOMY PROCEDURES

Both laminotomy and laminectomy procedures involve the removal of the **lamina** (the vertebral arch that protects the spinal cord) of one or more vertebra in order to reduce pressure on the spinal cord. The difference is the amount removed: laminotomies are partial, whereas a laminectomy removes the entire arch. There are several factors involved in coding these procedures. First, check the **section of the spine**, such as the cervical or lumbar, where the procedure is being performed. In addition, several codes are designed for only a single interspace. These codes will have add-on codes for additional interspaces that are covered by the procedure. For example, the laminotomy of three cervical interspaces would be covered by codes 63020 (for the first) and two instances of 63035 (for the other two interspaces).

SPINAL CORD

EXCISION OF INTRASPINAL LESIONS

An intraspinal lesion is a mass or tumor that is formed off the spinal cord or meninges and protrudes into the spinal canal. Treatment for intraspinal lesions is always surgical and may involve partial removal of the vertebral body. There are several factors that must be taken into consideration when selecting the proper codes for these procedures. First, check the **location of the lesion** that will be removed to determine whether it's **extradural** (outside the dura mater) or **intradural** (within the dura mater). Next, check the **location on the spine**: cervical, thoracic, lumbar, or sacral. Finally, check the **approach** that the surgeon or surgeons take to reach the lesion. Most of these codes are for a single segment, so if the surgery covers multiple segments, use the add-on code **63308** for each additional segment.

STEREOTACTIC RADIOSURGERY OF THE SPINE

Stereotactic radiosurgery is a type of specialized, nonsurgical radiation therapy used to inactivate or eradicate small tumors and other abnormalities within the brain and spinal cord, typically by applying precision doses of high-level radiation to the target. Codes in this section are used for the actual procedure. Treatment planning, dosimetry, and other treatment management by the oncologist can be found in codes **77261** through **77790**. These codes also include any planning,

42

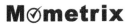

dosimetry, targeting, positioning, and blocking performed by the surgeon. It should be noted that the primary code, **63620**, should only be reported once, with the add-on code **63621** being reported once for each additional lesion, and only up to a maximum of twice regardless of the number of lesions treated.

EXTRACRANIAL, PERIPHERAL, AND AUTONOMIC NERVES

ANATOMICAL PURPOSES

This section of CPT covers three categories of nerves, each with their own part to play in the body: extracranial, peripheral, and autonomic nerves. Extracranial nerves are nerves that emerge from the skull, controlling and receiving signals to and from structures in the head, such as the eyes, ears, tongue, and nose. Peripheral nerves, meanwhile, are the nerves that branch off from the spinal cord and connect the central nervous system to the rest of the body, and they serve as sensors and to control the body's muscles (which are handled by **somatic nerves**) and organs. Finally, autonomic nerves are the parts of the peripheral nervous system that control the organs and glands involuntarily, allowing for the cardiovascular, respiratory, and digestive systems to operate without conscious input from the brain.

PROCEDURES

Procedures specifically involving extracranial, peripheral, and autonomic nerves are covered by CPT codes **64400** through **64913,** which are divided into subheadings based on the specific type of procedure. Procedures in this section include the following:

- Introduction and injection procedures to anesthetize nerves (known as **nerve blocks**)
- Implantation, revision, and replacement of neurostimulators
- Destruction of nerves via chemical and other means, particularly **chemodenervation**
- Surgical exploration and decompression of nerves and nerve tissue
- Transection or avulsion of nerves
- **Neurorrhaphy**, the surgical rejoining of split nerves, including the use of grafts.

These codes do not involve surgical intervention procedures on cranial nerves. For those procedures, see codes **61450, 61460,** and **61790.**

NERVE BLOCK

A nerve block is a procedure in which an anesthetic agent is injected into a nerve, nerve branch, or **nerve plexus** (a branching network of interlinked nerves) in order to block signals from a localized area for therapeutic or treatment purposes. There are several factors that must be accounted for when coding these procedures. First, check if **imaging guidance** is required or not because this will affect which type of code is used. Although most of the codes will have imaging guidance coded separately, some have it included in the procedure. Next, check **which nerve** is being injected. Finally, check **how many units or injections** are required by the code.

For further clarification, see the chart located in the "Introduction/Injection of Anesthetic Agent" subheading in this section of the CPT handbook.

NEUROPLASTY

Neuroplasty is a surgical procedure that is performed to relieve painful pressure on nerves, typically by removing scar tissue around the local area to free the nerve. A particularly common use of this is for the treatment of **carpal tunnel syndrome** (compression of the median nerve of the hand). Neuroplasty procedures can also include **neurolysis** (temporary artificial degeneration of nerve fibers), exploration, decompression, and transposition of nerve tissue. When coding these

43

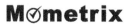

procedures, take note of the **anatomical location** of the nerve that is being treated and also any **additional procedures**, such as neurolysis or transposition, that are being performed as part of the procedure.

Eye and Ear

EYE/OCULAR ADNEXA
ANATOMICAL STRUCTURES

The eyes are the organs responsible for the collection and transmission of visual information to the brain, aka sight. The eyes are located in the curved **orbital** sections of the skull and consist of two sections: the **anterior** and **posterior**. The anterior section includes the **cornea**, the transparent covering of the front of the eye; the **iris**, the thin, muscle-controlled opening that forms the pupil; and the **lens**, the transparent, biconvex structure that focuses and refracts light. The posterior portion of the eye includes the jelly-like **vitreous humor** that fills the eye itself; the **retina**, which converts light into nerve signals; as well as the optic nerve. The eye is covered by the **sclera,** a whitish membrane that helps to protect the internal structures.

This section also covers the **adnexa**, or accessory structures of the eyes, including the muscles, the eyelids, and the **conjunctiva** (mucous membranes) and **lacrimal system** (tear-producing systems) that help lubricate them.

INTRAOCULAR LENS PROCEDURES

Intraocular lens procedures are procedures that involve the surgical removal and replacement of the lens, the part of the eye that focuses light on the retina. These procedures are typically performed to correct **cataracts**, a clouding and occlusion of the lens that typically occurs due to age or trauma. These procedures almost always include the insertion of a prosthetic lens to replace the damaged or diseased lens. There are several factors that must be accounted for when coding intraocular lens procedures. First, check whether the procedure is **extracapsular** or **intracapsular**, e.g., whether the tissue that covers the lens is left intact (extracapsular) or removed entirely (intracapsular). Next, check if the procedure includes **stages**. Most of the procedures are done in a single stage, but code **66985** is a two-stage procedure. In addition, take note of the parentheticals listed under some of the procedure descriptions for additional codes that may be needed to fully code the procedure.

SURGICAL PROCEDURES INVOLVING EXTRAOCULAR MUSCLES

The extraocular muscles are a set of five muscles that are attached to the eye, keeping it in place and allowing it to move around in its orbit. Surgical procedures involving the extraocular muscles typically involve the correction of **strabismus**, a condition in which one or both eyes remain out of alignment. As with most surgical procedures, there are several factors that must be taken into account when selecting the proper codes. First, check **which muscle** the procedure is being performed on. If the procedure is performed on the horizontal or vertical muscles, check the **number of muscles** (one or two) that the procedure is performed on. In addition, check for **prior surgeries or conditions** in this area, such as a detached extraocular muscle or a previous eye surgery.

AUDITORY SYSTEM
ANATOMICAL STRUCTURES

The auditory system is the body system responsible for capturing and transmitting sound-based stimuli to the brain, aka hearing. The auditory system is located on the head and includes the ears

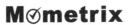

and related anatomical structures. The **ear**, which is the main auditory organ, is divided into three sections, the **outer**, **middle**, and **inner ear**. The outer ear is made up of the external cartilage and skin "funnel" of the **auricle**, the tube-like **external auditory canal** that leads to the fleshy **tympanic membrane**. The tympanic membrane forms the outer wall of the middle ear, which is made up of the **tympanic cavity** that contains the three bones of the ear, the **malleus**, **incus**, and **stapes**; as well as the **eustachian tube** that connects to the nasopharynx. The inner ear contains the **cochlea**, the spiral-shaped and fluid-filled structure that connects to the auditory nerve; as well as the hoop-like **semicircular canals** that help maintain balance. This area also includes parts of the temporal bones, the bones of the skull that the auditory system runs through.

TYMPANOPLASTY

A tympanoplasty is the surgical repair of a damaged or destroyed **tympanic membrane**. The tympanic membrane is the fleshy covering located at the end of the external auditory canal that protects and transmits sound to the tympanic cavity and is commonly referred to as the **eardrum**. There are a few factors that must be taken into account when coding tympanoplasty procedures. First, check which **other procedures are or are not included** along with the tympanic membrane, such as a mastoidectomy or an antrotomy. In addition, check whether or not an **ossicular chain reconstruction** is or is not included in the procedure because the associated codes are different from a standard tympanoplasty.

OPERATING MICROSCOPE

An operating microscope is a specialized type of microscope used by providers to visualize fine structures during a surgical procedure. This device is typically used for the purposes of conducting **microsurgery**, surgeries involving extremely small or delicate structures such as small nerves and tubes and parts of the ear, nose, and throat. Microsurgical techniques using an operating microscope are reported using code **69990**, which is an add-on code and cannot be reported individually. Do not report this code if magnifying loupes or corrected vision are used in the procedure. In addition, a large number of codes from multiple sections include the use of an operating microscope in their procedure codes and thus do not report this code separately. See the description of code 69990 for a full list of codes that include microsurgery using an operating microscope.

Evaluation and Management (E/M)

NEW AND ESTABLISHED PATIENTS

Codes for office and outpatient services are often divided by whether the patient is **new** or **established**. According to CPT guidelines, the criteria for new and established patients is determined by the following:

- A **new** patient is a patient who has not received any professional services from the physician or qualified healthcare professional in question, nor from a physician or qualified healthcare professional in the same group practice with the exact same specialty and subspecialty **within the past three years**.
- An **established** patient is a patient who has received professional services from the physician or qualified healthcare professional, or one in the same group practice with the exact same specialty and subspecialty within the past three years. This includes advanced practice nurses or physician assistants working with the physician or healthcare professional.

ROLE OF PATIENT'S HISTORY IN JUDGING AN E/M SERVICE ENCOUNTER

CPT divides a patient's **history** into three different parts: a **history of present illness**; a **review of symptoms by body system**; and the patient's **past, family, and social history**. A history of present illness covers the current issue, such as the location of the problem, the quality and severity of the symptoms, the timing and context of the symptoms, any modifying factors, and the duration. A review of symptoms covers what body systems are affected, including general constitution, eyes, ears, nose, mouth, throat, cardiovascular, respiratory, gastrointestinal, genitourinary, musculoskeletal, integumentary, neurological, psychiatric, endocrine, hematological, and allergic/immunological systems. Finally, past, family, and social history covers such issues as past health issues, family health issues, and issues such as tobacco and alcohol use. In general, the more factors that are mentioned in each category, the more comprehensive is the history.

EXAMINATION TYPES

Examinations refer to the physical or clinical inspection of a patient's affected areas or bodily systems. Types of examinations as defined by the American Academy of Professional Coders include the following:

- **Problem focused**, which is a limited examination of the problem site, area, or organ system
- **Expanded problem focused**, which includes the affected area and other symptomatic systems
- **Detailed**, which is an extended examination of the affected area and related or symptomatic systems
- **Comprehensive**, a general exam of multiple systems or a complete examination of a single organ system.

For the purposes of coding, CPT uses the following body areas and organ systems for examination: head (and face), neck, chest (and breasts and axilla), abdomen, genitalia (with the groin and buttocks), back, arms, legs, hands, feet, eyes, ears, nose, throat, mouth, cardiovascular system, respiratory system, gastrointestinal system, genitourinary system, musculoskeletal system, skin, neurological system, psychiatric, and hematological (and lymphatic and immunological).

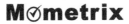

LEVELS OF MEDICAL DECISION MAKING

The level of medical decision making is how complex it is to establish a diagnosis and the management options. CPT categorizes medical decision making by using three factors: **management options**, **data**, and **risk of complications**. Management options are the number of possible treatment options available to treat the given issue. Data is the category that covers the complexity of medical records, diagnostic tests, and other information reviewed; the more difficult it is to access or analyze, the higher the complexity. Finally, the risk of complications involves how likely significant complications, such as a worsening condition or death, could occur in the course of treatment. These categories can be somewhat flexible, so care should be taken when assessing the procedure notes involving medical decision making.

SELECTION OF PROPER CATEGORIES FOR E/M SERVICES

Coding E/M services is difficult. Refer to the following charts for a simplified method of selecting the proper levels.

HISTORY

History of Present Illness	Review of Symptoms	Past, Family, and Social History	Level of History
Brief (1–3)	None	None	Problem focused
Brief (1–3)	1 body system	None	Expanded problem focused
Extended (4+)	2–9 body systems	1–2 of 3	Detailed
Extended (4+)	10–14 body systems	All	Comprehensive

EXAMINATION

Number of Systems or Areas Examined	Examination Type
Site of the problem only	Problem focused
Affected area and other symptomatic systems	Expanded problem focused
Extended examination of the affected area and related systems	Detailed
General exam or thorough exam of a single system	Comprehensive

MEDICAL DECISION MAKING

Management Options	Data	Risk of Complications	Level of Decision
1 (Minimal)	Minimal or none	Minimal	Straightforward
2 (Limited)	Limited	Low	Low complexity
3 (Multiple)	Moderate	Moderate (or prescription drugs)	Moderate complexity
4 (Extensive)	Extensive	High	High complexity

When selecting codes, code to the two lowest total levels of each category. For example, if a patient's history includes a brief history of present illness, a review of symptoms of two to nine body systems, and no history, then the history is problem focused. In medical decision making, the use of prescription drugs is always a moderate risk of complication.

ROLE OF TIME IN E/M PROCEDURES

Many E/M procedures will include a typical amount of time spent in face-to-face communication and interaction with the patient and/or their family. The time spent face to face with a patient is only a small factor when selecting the code needed for a procedure. However, if the provider spends

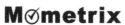

more than half of the total visit coordinating or counseling care, time may be used as a factor for selecting the proper code. For example, if an outpatient visit for an established patient has a detailed history, a detailed exam, and a high level of medical decision making (code 99213), but the practitioner takes 40 minutes counseling the patient, then the proper code would be 99215.

Place of Services

OFFICE AND OUTPATIENT SERVICES

Encounters for office and outpatient services are covered by codes **99201** through **99215** in CPT. Office and outpatient service codes are used to report E/M services in an office or outpatient facility. These services typically cover patients who visit a doctor's office or similar facilities and who are **ambulatory** (able to move under their own power) or suffering from relatively minor conditions. These typically include face-to-face services rendered by physicians and other qualified health professionals. Patients are considered outpatients until they are admitted to a healthcare facility, such as a hospital or nursing facility. These codes do not include emergency care.

CODING OUTPATIENT PROCEDURES

Outpatient admission codes require a history, examination, and a level of medical decision making to determine the proper codes. Refer to the following chart for a quick reference of the criteria for each code.

Code	History	Examination	Decision Making	Time
99201	Problem focused	Problem focused	Straightforward	10 min
99202	Expanded problem focused	Expanded problem focused	Straightforward	20 min
99203	Detailed	Detailed	Low	30 min
99204	Comprehensive	Comprehensive	Moderate	45 min
99205	Comprehensive	Comprehensive	High	60 min
99212	Problem focused	Problem focused	Straightforward	10 min
99213	Expanded problem focused	Expanded problem focused	Low	15 min
99214	Detailed	Detailed	Moderate	25 min
99215	Comprehensive	Comprehensive	High	40 min

New patients that are initially admitted for outpatient care will require three out of three components (history, examination, and medical decision making) to be listed. Established patients that are admitted for outpatient care require only two out of three components to be listed.

HOSPITAL OBSERVATION
OBSERVATION STATUS PROCEDURES

Observation status is a form of outpatient status that involves monitoring a patient for an extended period of time (typically one or more days) to determine if a patient must be admitted as an inpatient or if they can be safely discharged. Patients may be admitted for observation, in which case the initial observation care and subsequent observation care codes are used depending on the length of stay. If a patient is admitted for observation and then discharged on the same day, use codes **99234** through **99236**. If a patient under observation is admitted as an inpatient, then report the appropriate initial hospital admission code from **99221** through **99223**.

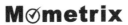

CODING OBSERVATION PROCEDURES

Observation codes require a history, examination, and a level of medical decision making to determine the proper codes. Refer to the following chart for a quick reference of the criteria for each code.

Code	History	Examination	Decision Making	Time
99218	Detailed	Detailed	Straightforward or low	30 min
99219	Comprehensive	Comprehensive	Moderate	50 min
99220	Comprehensive	Comprehensive	High	70 min
99224	Problem focused	Problem focused	Straightforward or low	15 min
99225	Expanded problem focused	Expanded problem focused	Moderate	25 min
99226	Detailed	Detailed	High	35 min

Patients (both new and established) who are admitted for observation will require three out of three components (history, examination, and medical decision making) to be listed. Each subsequent day of observation requires only two out of three components to be listed.

HOSPITAL INPATIENT

INPATIENT CARE PROCEDURES

Inpatient care is when a patient is admitted into a hospital or similar medical facility for the purposes of treatment. Inpatient care may last for one or more days, and it may be preceded by a period of observation. There are a few factors that may alter the use of inpatient care codes that should be accounted for. If the patient is 28 days old or younger (a neonate), then use code **99477** instead of an inpatient code. If the initial inpatient encounter is performed by someone other than the admitting physician, refer to codes **99251** through **99255** for consultation codes or **99231** through **99233** for subsequent hospital care codes. If the patient is admitted and discharged on the same day, refer to codes **99234** through **99236.**

CODING

Inpatient admission codes require a history, examination, and a level of medical decision making to determine the proper codes. Refer to the following chart for a quick reference of the criteria for each code.

Code	History	Examination	Decision Making	Time
99221	Detailed or comprehensive	Detailed or comprehensive	Straightforward or low	30 min
99222	Comprehensive	Comprehensive	Moderate	50 min
99223	Comprehensive	Comprehensive	High	70 min
99231	Problem focused	Problem focused	Straightforward or low	15 min
99232	Expanded problem focused	Expanded problem focused	Moderate	25 min
99233	Detailed	Detailed	High	35 min

Patients (both new and established) initially admitted for inpatient care will require three out of three components (history, examination, and medical decision making). Subsequent days of inpatient care require only two out of three components.

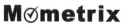

DISCHARGE SERVICE PROCEDURES

Discharge codes are used when a patient is cleared to leave the hospital after a period of observation and/or treatment. These codes include the final examination of a patient; discussion of the hospital stay; and preparation of any necessary referral forms, prescriptions, and discharge records. When coding, note the **amount of time** taken for the procedure because that determines which code is used. These codes are not to be used if the patient is admitted and discharged on the same day; if this occurs, see codes **99234** through **99236**. In addition, note the parentheticals underneath the code descriptions for additional contraindications and alternate codes.

CONSULTS

A consult is a form of E/M service that involves another physician, specialist, or other appropriate medical provider being brought in to assist the initial provider. Consulting providers may recommend care or procedures for specific issues or take over in the place of the initial provider. A consult is only coded if it is initiated by a physician or other appropriate source, not by the patient or their family. Consults may be performed in office/outpatient and inpatient settings. Procedures performed during or after the initial consult should be reported separately using the appropriate procedure codes. If the procedure is mandated by a third party, use modifier **32** in addition to the consult procedure code.

CODING

Consultation codes, both office-based and inpatient, require a history, examination, and a level of medical decision making to determine the proper codes. Refer to the following chart for a quick reference of the criteria for each code.

Code	History	Examination	Decision Making	Time
99241	Problem focused	Problem focused	Straightforward	15 min
99242	Expanded problem focused	Expanded problem focused	Straightforward	30 min
99243	Detailed	Detailed	Low	40 min
99244	Comprehensive	Comprehensive	Moderate	60 min
99245	Comprehensive	Comprehensive	High	80 min
99251	Problem focused	Problem focused	Straightforward	20 min
99252	Expanded problem focused	Expanded problem focused	Straightforward	40 min
99253	Detailed	Detailed	Low	55 min
99254	Comprehensive	Comprehensive	Moderate	80 min
99255	Comprehensive	Comprehensive	High	110 min

Consultations for patients (both new and established) will require three out of three components (history, examination, and medical decision making) in order to determine the proper code.

EMERGENCY DEPARTMENT

Emergency department services are E/M services that are used when a patient is admitted to the emergency department. CPT defines an emergency department as an organized, hospital-based facility for providing unscheduled episodic services, 24 hours a day, to patients requiring immediate medical care. Emergency department service codes also include a code for **directed emergency care** of ambulance or rescue personnel away from or en route to the hospital such as cardiac resuscitation, intubation of the airway, administration of intravenous fluids and injected drugs, and so on. Emergency department service codes do not cover services delivered during critical care.

PROCEDURES AND CODING

Emergency department codes require a history, examination, and a level of medical decision making to determine the proper codes. Refer to the following chart for a quick reference of the criteria for each code.

Code	History	Examination	Decision Making
99281	Problem focused	Problem focused	Straightforward
99282	Expanded problem focused	Expanded problem focused	Low
99283	Expanded problem focused	Expanded problem focused	Moderate
99284	Detailed	Detailed	Moderate
99285	Comprehensive	Comprehensive	High

Emergency department codes require three out of three components (history, examination, and medical decision making). Unlike other similar codes, time and whether the patient is new or established are not taken into account.

CRITICAL CARE

Critical care services are a type of E/M service used for direct delivery of medical care for a critically ill or injured patient by a qualified healthcare professional, often involving high-complexity decision making to assess and treat life-threatening deterioration or damage. This also covers transport of critically ill or injured patients to or from a hospital or other facility. The following services are included in critical care: interpreting cardiac output measurements, chest x-rays, pulse oximetry, blood gases, collection and interpretation of physiological data, temporary transcutaneous pacing, ventilatory management, and vascular access procedures. These codes only apply to patients 24 months of age and older; for younger patients, see codes **99471** through **99476.**

CODING

When coding critical care services, the patient history, examination, and medical decision making are disregarded. The key factor for critical care services is **time**; the primary code (**99291**) is for the first 30 to 74 minutes of service, whereas the add-on code **99292** is used for each additional 30-minute block. When coding these procedures, translate the given time into minutes and round up each 30-minute block. For example, a critical care service that lasts for 1 hour and 45 minutes would translate into 105 minutes, resulting in 99291 once and 99292 twice (74 + 30 + 1, which rounds up to 30).

Common codes included along with critical care services that are coded separately include CPR (**92950**), intubation (**31500**), and central line placement (**36620** through **36640, 36555, 36556,** and **36560**).

NURSING FACILITIES

Nursing facility services are E/M procedures used for patients in long-term care facilities, intermediate care facilities, and other convalescent or rehabilitative facilities. These facilities provide around-the-clock care for resident patients, often including a multidisciplinary plan of care. This also includes facilities that provide medical psychotherapy and similar treatments. These

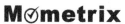

codes only cover medical care at the facility. For codes focused on care plan oversight for facility residents, see codes **99379** and **99380.** If a patient is admitted to a nursing facility in the process of an encounter at another site, such as a hospital, all of the E/M services provided in conjunction with that admission are considered part of the initial nursing facility care if they are performed on the same date. If a patient is discharged from inpatient status on the same date as admission or readmission to a nursing facility, use codes **99238** or **99239** as appropriate.

PROCEDURES AND CODING

Nursing facility care codes require a history, examination, and a level of medical decision making to determine the proper codes. Refer to the following chart for a quick reference of the criteria for each code.

Code	History	Examination	Decision Making	Time
99304	Detailed or comprehensive	Detailed or comprehensive	Straightforward or low	25 min
99305	Comprehensive	Comprehensive	Moderate	35 min
99306	Comprehensive	Comprehensive	High	45 min
99307	Problem focused	Problem focused	Straightforward or low	10 min
99308	Expanded problem focused	Expanded problem focused	Low	15 min
99309	Detailed	Detailed	Moderate	25 min
99310	Comprehensive	Comprehensive	High	35 min

Patients (both new and established) initially admitted to a nursing facility will require three out of three components (history, examination, and medical decision making). Subsequent days in the facility require only two out of three components.

DOMICILIARY AND REST HOMES

Domiciliary and rest home services are E/M procedures used for facilities that provide long-term care, room, board, and other personal assistance services to patients, typically elderly or otherwise infirm patients. These codes are used for assisted-living facilities, group homes, intermediate-care facilities, and other forms of custodial care facilities outside of the patient's home. It should be noted that the procedures coded in this section of CPT only cover E/M inside the facility. These codes only cover the E/M services provided, not the facility's actual services. For codes focused on care plan oversight for home health agencies, see codes **99374** and **99375.** For hospice agencies, see codes **99377** and **99378.**

PROCEDURES AND CODING

Domiciliary and rest home service codes require a history, examination, and a level of medical decision making to determine the proper codes. Refer to the following chart for a quick reference of the criteria for each code.

Code	History	Examination	Decision Making	Time
99324	Problem focused	Problem focused	Straightforward	20 min
99325	Expanded problem focused	Expanded problem focused	Low	30 min
99326	Detailed	Detailed	Moderate	45 min
99327	Comprehensive	Comprehensive	Moderate	60 min
99328	Comprehensive	Comprehensive	High	75 min
99334	Problem focused	Problem focused	Straightforward	15 min

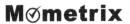

Code	History	Examination	Decision Making	Time
99335	Expanded problem focused	Expanded problem focused	Low	25 min
99336	Detailed	Detailed	Moderate	40 min
99337	Comprehensive	Comprehensive	High	60 min

Patients (both new and established) initially admitted to a rest home or domiciliary facility will require three out of three components (history, examination, and medical decision making). Subsequent days in the facility require only two out of three components.

HOME SERVICES

Home services are E/M procedures that are used when care is provided in the patient's own home. Home, as defined by CPT in this scenario, is referring to the patient's private residence, lodging, or short-term accommodations such as a hotel room. Home services may include doctor visits, at-home nursing care, home-based physical or occupational therapy, or other services rendered. These codes are used for E/M services only. For care plan oversight for a patient under the care of a home health agency, see codes **99374** and **99375,** or see codes **99377** and **99378** if oversight is provided by a hospice agency.

PROCEDURES AND CODING

Home service codes require a history, examination, and a level of medical decision making to determine the proper codes. Refer to the following chart for a quick reference of the criteria for each code.

Code	History	Examination	Decision Making	Time
99341	Problem focused	Problem focused	Straightforward	20 min
99342	Expanded problem focused	Expanded problem focused	Low	30 min
99343	Detailed	Detailed	Moderate	45 min
99344	Comprehensive	Comprehensive	Moderate	60 min
99345	Comprehensive	Comprehensive	High	75 min
99347	Problem focused	Problem focused	Straightforward	15 min
99348	Expanded problem focused	Expanded problem focused	Low	25 min
99349	Detailed	Detailed	Moderate	40 min
99350	Comprehensive	Comprehensive	High	60 min

New home care service patients will require three out of three components (history, examination, and medical decision making) to be listed. Established patients that are admitted for outpatient care require only two out of three components to be listed.

PREVENTATIVE MEDICINE

Preventative medicine covers E/M procedures meant for the evaluation of infants, children, adolescents, and adults without any issues or illness, such as annual physicals or well-woman exams. These services are meant to evaluate the overall health and well-being of the individual, as well as to identify any potential health problems before they fully manifest. These services include comprehensive history and examination, though not by the standards outlined by CPT as comprehensive. Preventative medicine services do not include things such as the administration of immunizations and vaccines, laboratory or radiology procedures, or screening tests identified with a specific CPT code; such services must be reported separately with the proper codes.

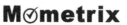

PROCEDURES AND CODING

Unlike many other E/M procedure codes, preventative medicine procedure codes do not require identifying the level of history, examination, and medical decision making. However, there are two major factors that must be taken into account. First, identify whether the patient is new or established because this is how the categories are initially divided. Second, check the **age** of the patient; procedure codes in this category are divided by patient age. These codes include counseling, anticipatory guidance, and risk reduction interventions provided during the procedure. If a problem is encountered but does not require additional work or require a problem-oriented E/M service, it should not be reported.

NON-FACE-TO-FACE SERVICES

TYPES

Non-face-to-face E/M services involve providers monitoring or reviewing patient status via long-distance methods, often without seeing patients directly. E/M services in this category include the following:

- **Telephone services**, in which qualified healthcare providers speak with patients or receive information over the phone
- **Online digital services**, which are patient-initiated services with a physician or qualified health provider over electronic communication such as secure email or electronic health records
- **Interprofessional consultations**, a type of consultation performed via telephone, Internet-based, or electronic health record services
- **Digitally stored data services** and **remote physiological monitoring**, in which remote devices (such as those in the patient's home) are interrogated for physiological data
- **Remote physiologic monitoring treatment management services**, in which the results from a remote monitoring device are used to manage a patient's treatment plan.

The devices used for these codes must be cleared by the Food and Drug Administration (FDA) before use, and all medical information transmitted must comply with HIPAA requirements.

CODING

Although non-face-to-face services encompass a wide variety of procedures and methodologies, many of them share similar factors that influence the selection of proper codes. A major component of these services, after the type of service is determined, is **time**. Each type of non-face-to-face E/M service, except digitally stored data services and remote physiological monitoring, requires a recorded amount of time in minutes, each having different ranges of time for each specific code. For digitally stored data services and remote physiological monitoring, code selection is based on the type of storage and device used for the data gathering, which is typically performed over 30-day periods.

NEONATAL AND PEDIATRIC CARE

NEWBORN CARE SERVICES

Newborn care services are E/M codes used for dealing with newborn children, which are defined by CPT as an age range from birth through the first 28 days. These codes include services such as maternal and fetal history, physical examinations of the newborn, ordering of diagnostic tests and treatments, family meetings, and documentation. These codes cover care, not procedures performed on newborns (such as circumcision). Those codes are reported separately to the care service codes. If a newborn patient is later admitted for intensive care or additional critical care on

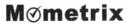

the same day that one of these codes is used, report the appropriate E/M code for the admission with modifier 25 alongside the newborn service code.

DELIVERY/BIRTHING ROOM ATTENDANCE AND RESUSCITATION SERVICES

The "Newborn Care Services" section also includes delivery/birthing room attendance and resuscitation services, in which a doctor or other qualified health professional is in attendance and present at the birth to provide the initial stabilization of the newborn. This code, **99464**, is used in conjunction with other related codes such as 99460.

This section also includes the code if the aforementioned health professional is required to perform CPR on a newborn postdelivery in the event of inadequate cardiac or respiratory output. Other procedures for resuscitation, such as intubation, are reported separately. This code, **99465**, is not reported in conjunction with 99464; it supersedes that one when it is used.

INTENSIVE CARE
CODING INPATIENT NEONATAL AND PEDIATRIC CRITICAL CARE SERVICES

Inpatient neonatal and pediatric critical care service codes are used when a critically ill **neonate** (a child aged 28 days old or younger) or a **pediatric** (a child aged 29 days old or older) patient is put into the pediatric intensive care unit or the neonatal intensive care unit. The codes in this section are divided by age: 28 days or younger, 29 days to 24 months, and 2 to 5 years old. A variety of codes are included in this section, including the following: vascular access procedures, airway and ventilation management, monitoring/interpretation of blood gases and oxygen saturation, car seat evaluation, transfusion of blood components, oral or nasogastric tube placement, suprapubic bladder aspiration, bladder catheterization, and lumbar puncture. All other services should be reported separately.

CODING CONTINUING INTENSIVE CARE SERVICES FOR NEONATES

The use of initial and continuing intensive care service E/M codes is intended for neonates and infants who are not critically ill but still require intensive observation, intervention, and continuing care. These are typically used for premature newborns or newborn children with a low birth weight. These services include vital sign monitoring, heat maintenance, nutritional adjustments, and observation by a healthcare team directed by a physician. Procedures listed for neonatal and pediatric critical care codes are also bundled with these codes, and they should not be reported separately. These codes are reported once per day, unless the neonate or infant's condition improves to the point that intensive care is no longer required.

PROLONGED SERVICES

Prolonged services are E/M procedures in which a physician or other qualified healthcare provider performs prolonged or extended service or services beyond what is typically required in an inpatient or outpatient setting. Such services are reported in addition to the primary procedure and cover procedures that are performed with direct patient contact, without direct patient contact, or involving clinical staff or other qualified healthcare professional supervision. These codes only apply to E/M services or psychotherapy services: Other services that are provided are not counted toward the prolonged services. Any medications or supplies used or additional procedures performed during the prolonged services should be coded alongside the prolonged services codes.

CODING

There are several factors to take into consideration when coding prolonged E/M services. The first and most obvious factor is the **type of service.** Prolonged services codes cover procedures that are performed with direct patient contact, without direct patient contact, or involving clinical staff or other qualified healthcare professional supervision. The next most important factor is the **time spent**. Codes in this section are selected based on the amount of time spent (calculated in minutes), with multiple codes being required to indicate longer amounts of time. For example, if the total duration of a prolonged service with direct contact is 77 minutes, the codes used would be **99354** and **99355**. Also, prolonged services of less than a minimum level (30 minutes for direct and no direct contact, 45 minutes for supervised) are not separately reported. These codes are add-on codes, so do not report them on their own.

CHRONIC CARE

Chronic care services are E/M procedures in which a physician or other qualified healthcare provider offers the establishment, implementation, revision, or monitoring of a care plan designed to handle two or more chronic health conditions when the medical or psychosocial needs of the patient require them. These conditions may be continuous or episodic issues that are expected to last at least 12 months or until the death of the patient. In addition, the condition or conditions should place the patient at significant risk of exacerbation, decline, or death. These codes cover management of both standard and complex care management. **Complex** care management refers to chronic issues requiring multiple specialties and those that limit daily activities, complicate care, or require social support.

CODING

Coding chronic care procedures requires certain elements in order to qualify. These include the following, as laid out by CPT guidelines:

- There are multiple chronic conditions that last for 12 months or until the death of the patient.
- The conditions place the patient at a significant risk of death, acute exacerbation, or decline.
- A comprehensive care plan is established, implemented, revised, and/or monitored.

In addition, complex care management has two additional criteria:

- Moderate- or high-complexity medical decision making
- 60 minutes of clinical staff time per calendar month directed by a qualified healthcare professional or performed by a physician.

Both categories are coded based on the **amount of time** of the encounter. Complex services have much longer time allotments, and the add-on code **99489** should be used for every 30-minute block after the initial 60 minutes. For example, a complex care service that lasts for 99 minutes uses codes 99487 and 99489 once (60 + 39, rounded down to 30).

TRANSITIONAL CARE

Transitional care services are E/M procedures involving the transition of a patient with medical or psychosocial problems from an inpatient hospital setting (acute or long term), partial hospital setting, observation, or skilled nursing facility to a community setting (such as the patient's home, a rest home, or an assisted living facility). These patients must have issues requiring a moderate to high level of medical decision making (as defined by CPT). These services include at least one face-to-face visit within the specified timeframe, any additional non-face-to-face services performed by the physician or qualified healthcare professional and/or clinical staff, and coordination of care between multiple disciplines.

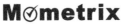

CODING

Coding transitional care procedures requires certain elements in order to qualify. These include the following, as laid out by CPT guidelines:

- Communication in the form of direct, electronic, or telephone contact between the patient or patient's caregiver within 2 business days of discharge
- Medical decision making of moderate (for code **99495**) or high (for code **99496**) complexity within the service period
- A face-to-face visit within 7 (for code **99496**) or 14 (for code **99495**) calendar days after the date of discharge.

Procedures of this type involving high complexity only use code **99496** for the face-to-face visit within 7 days. All other instances of transitional care that involve face-to-face visits within 8 to 14 days use code **99495**, regardless of the complexity of medical decision making. Do not report these codes in conjunction with codes **93792** or **93793**.

CASE MANAGEMENT

Case management services are the E/M procedures that are used when a physician or other qualified healthcare professional is directly caring for and initiating, coordinating, managing, or supervising additional healthcare services needed by the patient. This often involves conferences, either face-to-face or indirectly, between the physician, their team of healthcare professionals, and the patient and their family. When coding these procedures, the codes separate nonphysician qualified healthcare professionals from physicians: If a face-to-face conference with the patient is performed by the overseeing physician, that physician reports using the appropriate E/M procedure code.

CARE PLAN OVERSIGHT

Care plan oversight services are E/M procedures that cover recurrent supervision of a patient by a physician or other skilled healthcare provider. These codes are used for the supervision of multidisciplinary care in home healthcare environments, hospices, or nursing facilities. Such services include review of care plans and laboratory reports, communication with healthcare professionals, family members, legal guardians and caregivers, modification or adjustment of medical treatment plans, and adjustment of medical therapy. These codes are divided by location of the patient and the time involved in the actual act of supervision. Care plan oversight of assisted-living facilities or hospice agencies use codes separate from these.

Anesthesia

TIME REPORTING

Anesthesia time refers to the amount of time that an individual is placed under anesthesia for a procedure in the operating room or an equivalent area. During this time, the patient is under the care of the **anesthesiologist**, a medical professional specially trained in the administration of anesthetics. Procedures involving anesthesia will have an amount of time listed, either in whole or in part, as part of the procedure notes. As outlined by CPT, anesthesia time begins with the time it takes the anesthesiologist to prepare the patient for the induction of anesthesia and it ends when the anesthesiologist is officially no longer in personal attendance.

PROCEDURES INCLUDED OR CODED SEPARATELY FROM ANESTHESIA PROCEDURES

Anesthesia procedure codes include a variety of additional services that will likely be used during the administration and monitoring of an anesthetized patient. These services are performed under the supervision of the physician in charge, and they vary widely. These include the use of supplementation of local anesthesia; preoperative and postoperative visits; anesthesia care during the actual procedure; the administration of fluid and/or blood; as well as forms of monitoring such as temperature, blood pressure, oximetry, electrocardiogram, capnography, and others. Some unusual forms of monitoring may also be used, including intra-arterial catheters (**36629** and **36625**), central venous pressure (**36655** and **36656**), Swan-Ganz catheters (**93503**), and endotracheal intubation (**31500**). These unusual services are coded separately.

QUALIFYING CIRCUMSTANCES

Qualifying circumstance codes are used when anesthesia must be administered under extreme or otherwise difficult circumstances based on the condition of the patient or the circumstances of the operation. These may include extreme age (young or old); the requirement of **full-body hypothermia** (cooling the body down to a very low temperature); the use of **controlled hypotension** (artificially lowering blood pressure); or conditions that would mean significant threat to the patient's life, health, or body parts if there's a delay. Qualifying circumstance codes are all add-on codes, meaning they are used in conjunction with anesthesia codes and cannot be coded on their own.

GENERAL AND MONITORED ANESTHESIA CARE

Anesthesia is typically divided into two different categories based on the intended outcome. For **general anesthesia**, a patient is placed into a sleep-like state of unconsciousness for the duration of the operation and is brought out of it during recovery. **Conscious sedation**, also known as **moderate sedation** or **monitored anesthesia care (MAC)**, is a form of anesthesia in which the patient remains conscious enough to follow instructions but is generally calm and unable to feel pain. When coding anesthesia procedures that use the phrase "requires anesthesia," assume that the procedure is using MAC unless general anesthesia is explicitly mentioned.

PHYSICAL STATUS MODIFIERS

Physical status modifiers are modifiers, appended after an anesthesia code, that indicate the general level of health or status of the patient undergoing anesthesia. These modifiers are listed as P1 through P6 and are mandatory unless the billing is performed through Medicare. The modifiers are consistent with the guidelines established by the American Society of Anesthesiologists for ranking physical status, and they include the following:

- **P1:** A healthy patient
- **P2:** A patient with a mild systemic disease
- **P3:** A patient with a severe systemic disease
- **P4:** The same as P3, but the disease is a constant threat to life
- **P5:** A patient that is not expected to survive without the operation
- **P6:** A declared brain-dead patient whose organs are being removed for donation.

COMMON HCPCS MODIFIERS USED FOR ANESTHESIA CODES

Anesthesia procedure codes may require additional modifiers depending on the circumstances surrounding the procedure. These modifiers are appended to the end of a procedure code when applicable, and are typically used for MAC during a surgical procedure. These codes are not always required for every procedure; they are required for atypical circumstances, such as when a procedure has to end before completion or if unusual methods must be used. Common HCPCS modifiers include the following:

- **23:** Unusual anesthesia
- **47:** Anesthesia performed by surgeon
- **53:** Discontinued procedure (in this case, meaning the anesthesia itself is discontinued)
- **59:** Distinct procedural service
- **73:** Discontinued outpatient procedure prior to anesthesia administration
- **74:** Discontinued outpatient procedure subsequent to anesthesia administration.

HCPCS LEVEL II MODIFIERS

These modifiers, found in the HCPCS book, are some of the most commonly used modifiers for anesthesia procedures. These alphabetical and alphanumeric codes are typically used for MAC during a surgical procedure, and they help to properly describe the procedure as presented. Several of these codes are used when one or more certified registered nurse anesthetists (CRNAs) are involved in the procedure. These codes include the following:

- **AA**: Anesthesia performed personally by an anesthesiologist
- **AD:** Medical supervision by a physician of more than four concurrent anesthesia procedures
- **G8:** MAC for deep, complex, or highly invasive procedures
- **G9**: MAC for severe cardiopulmonary condition
- **QK**: Medical direction of two to four concurrent anesthesia procedures
- **QS**: MAC service
- **QX:** CRNA service without medical direction by an anesthesiologist
- **QY**: One CRNA service directed by an anesthesiologist
- **QZ**: CRNA service without direction by a physician.

ANESTHESIA FOR SERVICES

ANESTHESIA CODES FOR SURGICAL PROCEDURES

The majority of codes in CPT's "Anesthesia" section cover procedures involving anesthesia for various types of surgical procedures. Codes in the "Anesthesia" section are divided primarily by anatomical location. It should be noted that, unless the anesthetic procedure code includes an actual description of a specific type of procedure (e.g., "Anesthesia for all closed procedures on lower leg, ankle, or foot"), the code description will typically include the phrase "**Not otherwise**

specified," meaning that it covers a broad category of procedures. These codes will often have additional codes listed underneath to help indicate a more specific code, such as "Repair of ruptured Achilles tendon, with or without graft." When possible, select the most precise code for the procedure given.

ANESTHESIA CODES FOR DIAGNOSTIC PROCEDURES

Several codes in CPT's "Anesthesia" section cover anesthesia for various types of diagnostic procedures. As with surgical codes, the majority of these procedures are grouped by anatomical location. When selecting codes for a diagnostic procedure, check the code description and give the procedure description for the proper terms used. Diagnostic procedures will include terms such as:

- Diagnostic
- Biopsy (such as percutaneous liver biopsy)
- Screening (such as screening colonoscopy)
- Procedures that end with the suffixes "-scopy" or "-graphy," such as arthroscopy or cholangiopancreatography.

As noted in the "Surgery" sections of CPT, most surgical procedures will have a diagnostic portion included in their procedure code. This should be kept in mind when coding anesthesia for diagnostic procedures: Only code using anesthesia for a diagnostic procedure when a separate diagnostic procedure is being performed.

ANESTHESIA CODES FOR RADIOLOGICAL PROCEDURES

Certain radiological procedures may require the use of anesthesia depending on the patient's health or condition. Radiological procedures mentioned in the "Anesthesia" section of CPT include the following:

- Diagnostic arteriography and venography
- Cardiac catheterization
- Radiation therapy
- Radiological intervention in the arterial, venous, or lymphatic systems
- Percutaneous, image-guided procedures on the spine and spinal cord.

Note the specific anatomical area that the radiological procedure is being performed on because that will influence which anesthesia code is selected for the procedure if required. These codes may or may not be included in the procedure code for the radiological procedure in question; read through the procedure code description before adding more codes.

ANESTHESIA CODES FOR OBSTETRIC PROCEDURES

Certain obstetric procedures may require the use of anesthesia depending on the procedure or the patient's health status. Many of the codes involved in this section of anesthesia will cover anesthesia involved in delivery, including the following:

- Vaginal delivery
- Cesarean
- Hysterectomy, either following delivery or without labor
- Incomplete, missed, or induced abortions
- Neuraxial labor anesthesia, typically through an epidural catheter, during or in preparation for labor.

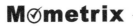

Some of these codes (**01968** and **01969**) are add-on codes used in conjunction with earlier codes in this section. When coding these anesthesia procedures, confirm the primary procedure that is associated with the anesthesia code.

Radiology

RADIOLOGICAL PROCEDURES

Radiological procedures are procedures that involve the use of various imaging techniques to diagnose and treat illnesses, often by using some form of directed energy. Radiological procedures cover a variety of methodologies that are used to observe internal body structure, including **ultrasound**, which uses high-frequency sound waves; **x-rays**, which use x-ray radiation; and **magnetic resonance imaging**, or **MRI**, which uses magnetic fields and radio waves. This section also includes **nuclear medicine**, which is when carefully measured traces of radioactive substances are used to locate, diagnose, and treat diseases. These procedures can be performed either separately as individual services, or in tandem with other procedures for the purposes of visualization or treatment.

PROCEDURES IN "RADIOLOGY" SECTION OF CPT

Radiological procedures are covered by codes **70010** through **79999** in the CPT book, which are divided into related headings and subheadings throughout the section. Procedures in this section include the following:

Diagnostic radiology	Examination of body structures via radiological methods such as x-ray or MRI
Diagnostic ultrasound	Examination of various body structures via high-frequency sound waves
Radiological guidance	Radiological methods are used in conjunction with other procedures to guide treatment
Mammography	Radiological inspection of the mammary glands
Bone and joint studies	Includes bone densitometry and joint radiography
Radiation oncology	High-dose radiation of various sources used to treat cancer
Nuclear medicine	Radioactive substances introduced to the body to locate and diagnose disease

DIAGNOSTIC RADIOLOGY
CONTRAST MATERIALS

Many diagnostic radiology procedures include one of two phases: **without contrast material** or **with contrast material.** A contrast material is a substance, often injected, consumed, or otherwise introduced into the body, that has a different opacity from the surrounding soft tissue when viewed radiologically. When a procedure uses contrast material in a radiological procedure, introduced via injection either into a vein, a joint, or the spinal canal, it uses a different CPT code. It should be noted, however, that if a contrast material is only administered orally (via the mouth) or rectally (via the rectum), then the procedure is technically considered "without contrast" for the purposes of coding the procedure.

VASCULAR DIAGNOSTIC PROCEDURES

Vascular diagnostic procedures are when a contrast material is injected into a major artery, vein, or lymphatic vessel in order to properly view them to diagnose issues. These procedure codes are not to be used with interventional procedures because they are meant for diagnostic purposes alone, and intervention codes already bundle these services in. There are several factors to consider when

62

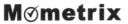

coding these types of procedures. In addition to defining the **type of vessel being viewed** (such as an artery or vein), one must take into account the **area being viewed**, such as an extremity. It is also important to check the **laterality** of the exam, i.e., whether it's unilateral or bilateral.

DIAGNOSTIC ULTRASOUND
PROCEDURES AND CODING

Diagnostic ultrasounds are radiological procedures that use ultra-high frequency sound waves emitted and recorded by specialized machines to visualize a body's internal structures to examine and diagnose issues. These procedures cover a variety of soft tissues, including the circulatory system. When coding these procedures, they may include a number of different scans, including an **A-mode** scan, a simple measurement of an echo to determine depth; a **B-mode** scan, a static two-dimensional image generated by sound; an **M-mode** scan, a recorded two-dimensional image in motion; or a real-time two-dimensional scan with motion.

OBSTETRIC ULTRASOUND PROCEDURES

Ultrasound imaging is commonly used for obstetric purposes, typically to visualize and document the fetus or fetuses for evaluation during gestation. Most codes involving these include real-time image documentation. There are several factors that must be taken into account when coding these procedures. First, check the **approach** used for the procedure, whether it's transabdominal or transvaginal. Next, check what else is **documented** during the procedure, such as an examination of the fetus's anatomy or the fetal heartbeat. In addition, check for any **additional factors** that would affect the code selection, such as the trimester or number of fetuses. Finally, if the procedure is not an ultrasound, check what other factors are involved before selecting a final code.

RADIOLOGICAL GUIDANCE PROCEDURES

Radiological guidance procedures are when a radiological method, such as **fluoroscopy** (a type of x-ray that captures real-time movement of internal structures), **computed tomography** (a computerized x-ray that captures cross-sectional images of the body and its organs), or MRI is used to help guide surgical or other treatments such as biopsies or tissue ablation. These procedures are divided by method of visualization, and they are often accompanied by a list of codes that are used either in conjunction with or to avoid being reported with. When coding these procedures, it's extremely important to **check the parentheticals** in order to see whether or not the procedure code is reported separately from the procedure it provides guidance for. Several codes in the "Surgery" sections of CPT have these codes bundled in with the procedure.

MAMMOGRAPHY

Mammograms are a specific type of radiological procedure that involves scanning the breasts for masses or lesions within the soft tissue. These procedures often involve a specialized scanning device that helps flatten the mass of the breast to improve the quality of the image. There are several factors that must be accounted for when coding these procedures. First, check the **specific procedure** being performed, such as a digital breast tomosynthesis or a mammogram. If the procedure is a mammogram, check whether the procedure is **diagnostic** or **screening**. Generally speaking, screening mammography is a routine procedure, whereas diagnostic mammography is used when a problem is suspected. Furthermore, check the **laterality** of the procedure, e.g., whether it's a unilateral or bilateral procedure.

BONE AND JOINT STUDIES

Radiological procedures involving the study of bones and joints are typically performed to study the density or shape of the bones or joints being scanned or to assess fractures, particularly of the vertebrae. There are a few factors that must be taken into account when coding these procedures.

First, determine the **procedure** being performed. Next, check which **parts of the skeleton** are being scanned, if applicable. Certain procedures may call for a **dual-energy X-ray absorptiometry** scan, a type of bone density imaging that uses two x-ray beams of differing energy levels. For these procedures, only report a single procedure code, no matter how many sites are scanned.

RADIATION ONCOLOGY

Radiation oncology is a set of radiological procedures that use carefully controlled high-intensity radiation from various sources to carefully treat or eliminate diseased or cancerous tissue in the body. Like other therapeutic treatments, radiation oncology procedure codes include related services such as the initial consultation, simulation of the procedure, dosimetry, clinical treatment management and planning procedures and other special services, as well as normal follow-up care during treatment and in the three months after the completion of treatment. These codes do not cover preliminary consultation, the evaluation of the patient, or additional care provided by the radiologist because those events use different codes from different sections of CPT.

TREATMENT PLANNING

Radiation treatment planning procedures cover the services involved in setting up a radiation treatment, such as interpretation of tests; determination of treatment time, dosage, and volume; and choice of modality. These codes are labeled as simple, intermediate, or complex in the procedural description in order to define the planning and simulation used in the procedure. **Simple** refers to a single treatment area, either for planning or simulation; **intermediate** refers to two separate treatment areas, often requiring three or more ports or multiple blocks; and **complex** involves three or more separate treatment areas, often including very complex blocking, compensation, or specialized treatment modality.

RADIATION TREATMENT DELIVERY

Radiation treatment delivery procedures cover the actual administration of radiation during radiation oncology. These methods include x-rays, intensity-modulated radiation therapy (IMRT), electron beams, neutron beams, and proton beams. Similar to planning procedures, delivery procedures are labeled as simple, intermediate, or complex when describing procedures. **Simple** codes cover a single treatment area; one or two ports or blocks; or IMRT of the breasts, prostate, or sites needing a physical compensator. **Intermediate** codes cover treatment of two separate areas, three or more ports, or simple blocks. **Complex** codes cover three or more areas; custom blocking, wedges, or additional compensation; or IMRT that doesn't use a physical compensator.

CLINICAL BRACHYTHERAPY PROCEDURES

Clinical brachytherapy is a form of radiation oncology that uses implanted radioelements, natural and artificial, to treat cancerous tissue. These implants are divided into two types: **sources,** which are permanently placed interstitially or inside a cavity; or **ribbons**, which are temporary implants. Like other radiation oncology procedures, brachytherapy uses a category system of simple, intermediate, and complex when describing procedures. **Simple** refers to the placement of 1 to 4 elements, **intermediate** refers to the placement of 5 to 10 elements, and **complex** applications are when more than 10 elements are placed within the body. When coding these procedures, always note the **dose rate** and any **channels** that are mentioned in the procedure description.

NUCLEAR MEDICINE PROCEDURES

Nuclear medicine procedures are radiological services that involve the introduction of radioactive tracer substances into the body, either inhaled, injected into the bloodstream, or ingested, to locate and diagnose diseases in various bodily systems. These types of procedures can be performed separately or in tandem with other procedures. These procedures do not include the actual

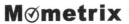

radiopharmaceuticals (the radioactive substances used for the procedure) and drugs used in the procedure: When coding these procedures, include the supply code for the substances used. In addition, confirm the areas and types of imaging performed in the procedure's description.

CARDIOVASCULAR SYSTEM

Typical nuclear medicine procedures performed on the cardiovascular system include **myocardial perfusion**, in which radioactive tracer substances flow through the blood that supplies the cardiac muscle; and **cardiac blood pool imaging**, which tracks how blood flows through the heart to the rest of the body. Several factors may impact the coding of these procedures. First, check the **type of procedure** performed, as usual. Next, check the **type of technique or scan** (such as a single-photon emission computerized tomography test or a first-pass technique) that is performed. In addition, note the **number of studies** performed during the procedure because multiple studies can be performed during a single procedure.

Laboratory and Pathology

LABORATORY AND PATHOLOGY PROCEDURES

Laboratory and pathology procedures cover various types of diagnostic lab work used in the diagnosis of diseases and conditions. This section covers codes **80047** through **89398** and **0001U** through **0061U** and contains the following procedures:

- Organ and disease-oriented panels
- Drug assays, both therapeutic and nontherapeutic
- Consultations on clinical pathology
- Urinalysis (testing urine)
- Molecular pathology (analysis of genetic material)
- Genomic sequencing
- Hematology and coagulation studies (testing blood)
- Immunology studies
- Transfusion medicine (tests used on donor blood)
- Microbiology studies (analysis of bacteria, viruses, and similar specimens)
- Anatomical and surgical pathology (inspecting cells and tissue taken from patients)
- Cytopathology and cytogenetic studies
- Reproductive medicine procedures
- Specialist and proprietary lab analysis procedures.

ORGAN AND DISEASE PANELS

Organ and disease panels are a type of procedure that analyzes and quantifies various chemicals and substances in a blood sample to provide information on metabolic functions and physical status. Each type of panel tests a number of different substances, such as albumin, glucose, potassium, sodium, urea nitrogen, and antibodies. When coding these procedures, it is important to select the code that contains as many substances listed in the procedure description as possible. If there's an overlap between two types of panels, choose the one that includes the largest number of listed substances and code the remainder as individual tests. In addition, pay attention to the specific substances listed in each panel because they may differ between similar panels. For instance, calcium is included in two types of basic metabolic panels, but one uses ionized calcium whereas the other uses total calcium.

DRUG TESTING

TYPES OF DRUG TESTING PROCEDURES

Drug assays are procedures used to detect the presence of drugs in the patient or subject's body, typically through blood, urine, or other bodily fluids or tissues. Drug assays are divided into two different types: **presumptive** and **definitive**. A presumptive drug procedure is used to identify the possible presence of a drug or a general class of drug in the subject's body. Meanwhile, a definitive drug procedure is used to determine a qualitative and/or quantitative value of a drug in the patient's system. It should be noted that, although both tests are often performed in sequence, a definitive test does not by definition require a presumptive test. Also, if the same type of procedure is performed on multiple specimen types from a single patient, then modifier 59 should be used in conjunction with the appropriate codes.

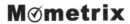

PRESUMPTIVE DRUG CLASS SCREENING

Presumptive drug class screening procedures are used to identify the possible presence of a drug or a general class of drug in the subject's body. There are a few factors that must be taken into account when coding these types of procedures. The primary factor that defines the code selected is the **method of analysis**, whether by direct observation, such as a card or dipstick; or by chemical analysis, such as chromatography or mass spectrometry. These codes are only reported once, regardless of how many classes of drugs are tested for. Always check the procedure notes to determine what types of processes are used.

DEFINITIVE DRUG TESTING

Definitive drug testing procedures are used to identify specific classes of drugs, both in type and number, in a given patient's system. This process typically covers in-depth analysis, such as chromatography with mass spectrometry. The primary factor that defines the code selected is the **class of drug**, such as alcohols or skeletal muscle relaxants. An additional factor for some codes is the **number of analytes**. For example, the code for three or more alcohol biomarkers is different from just one. Although some codes are meant for specific drugs, such as cocaine, other codes cover a generic class. For example, the drugs Paxil, Prozac, and Doxepin would fall under code 80335 because they're all cyclic antidepressants.

THERAPEUTIC DRUG ASSAYS

Therapeutic drug assays are a type of drug testing procedure used to measure the presence and quantity of a specific prescribed medicine in the patient's system. This is done to monitor the levels of medical substances in order to keep the amount of drug within therapeutic levels and to prevent overdose or otherwise toxic side effects. This is typically performed on blood, blood serum, blood plasma, or CSF. These procedures are coded based on the **specific drug**, similar to definitive drug testing. Unlike definitive drug testing, the number of metabolites or other units is not required to be known for code selection purposes.

EVOCATIVE/SUPPRESSION TESTING

MEDICAL PURPOSE

Evocative/suppression testing is a form of laboratory procedure designed to measure the release of certain bodily substances, enzymes, and hormones, such as corticotropin-releasing hormone or insulin. During the test, a particular enzyme, hormone, or other bodily substance is given an initial measurement. Then, additional substances are administered in order to elicit a response to determine if the levels are either suppressed or stimulated, after which the measurements are repeated and quantified. These procedures are often repeated multiple times.
Evocative/suppression testing is typically performed to test for disorders of the endocrine system, such as human growth hormone deficiency, renal problems, or thyroid issues.

CODING

Evocative/suppression testing covers the laboratory procedures involved in the testing of certain bodily substances, enzymes, and hormones. Similar to organ and disease panels, each code includes multiple types of substance that are tested, although evocative/suppression tests typically have multiple iterations of each test. For example, an aldosterone suppression panel has two instances of aldosterone and two renin analyses. However, the individual tests themselves are not coded, so an aldosterone suppression panel would only use the single code 80408 as opposed to the four individual codes for the tests used. When reviewing the procedure notes, make sure that all iterations of each substance are mentioned and accounted for. These codes are for the actual testing procedure; for the administration of the actual evocative or suppressive substances, see codes

67

96365 through **96368** and **96372** through **96376** located in the "Medicine" section of the CPT handbook.

CONSULTATIONS

A clinical pathology consult is when a physician or other qualified healthcare provider requests the services, including written reports or information of the movement of drugs within the body, of a clinical pathologist in relation to tests and professional judgment. These procedures are distinct from a standard E/M consult because they do not involve the pathologist evaluating the patient. This does not include simply reporting test results. When coding these procedures, confirm whether the consultation did or did not include a **review of the patient's history and records** because that defines the complexity of the consult. If the consult includes evaluating or examining a patient, see the relevant codes in the "E/M" section of CPT.

URINALYSIS

Urinalysis is a set of laboratory procedures that revolve around the testing of a patient's urine. Although urinalysis is used in other procedures such as drug tests, the codes in the "Urinalysis" section of CPT focus on separately identifiable procedures, typically testing for substances in the urine such as glucose, hemoglobin, and protein; screening and culture of bacteria; or pregnancy tests that use urine. When coding these procedures, check the procedure notes for the specific **purpose** of the test. In addition, if the test is performed to check for substances, check the level of **automation** and the use of **microscopy**. If a specific analysis is being performed, refer to the appropriate subsection of the "Pathology and Laboratory" section.

MOLECULAR PATHOLOGY

PROCEDURES AND CODES

Molecular pathology covers a number of laboratory procedures involving the analysis of deoxyribonucleic acid (DNA) and ribonucleic acid in order to detect for various genetic disorders and related issues. This is done by analyzing a patient's genetic code for **germline** or **somatic** variations to see if the patient's genes do not match the normal sequence. Germline variations are inherited genetics, whereas somatic variations are singular mutations that aren't passed down. This section also includes tests for **human leukocyte antigens**, which are the protein markers that help regulate the immune system. Codes in this section include all of the analytic services involved in performing the tests, and they are divided into tiers based on how commonly the procedure is performed.

TIER 1 MOLECULAR PATHOLOGY PROCEDURES

Tier 1 molecular pathology procedures are a set of molecular pathology procedures from **81170** through **81383** that are commonly performed. These codes represent gene-specific procedures that cover a wide variety of common genetic disorders, such as fragile X syndrome, cystic fibrosis, sickle cell anemia, hereditary nonpolyposis colorectal cancer, and other issues. Procedure codes are defined by the specific sequence, or **analyte**, that they cover, and they include a list of **associated disorders** or conditions that are being tested for. Several codes will focus on a **specific type of analysis**. For example, 81223 is a full gene sequence analysis cystic fibrosis transmembrane conductance regulator. When reviewing the procedure notes for these codes, check for any other details of the analysis that may be mentioned.

TIER 2 MOLECULAR PATHOLOGY PROCEDURES

Tier 2 molecular pathology procedures list a variety of molecular pathology procedures that are uncommon or rare compared to the procedures listed in Tier 1. Although medically necessary, the procedures used are performed at lower rates due to a relative scarcity of the disease being tested

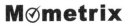

for. Unlike Tier 1 procedures, Tier 2 procedures are grouped by the **level** of analysis required, like a Level 7 procedure that covers an 11 to 25 exon DNA sequence analysis, as well as the specific sequence being analyzed. Each code covers a wide variety of analysis procedure, listed alphabetically by analyte, so procedure notes should always be checked for the specific procedure. If the specific analyte is not covered by either Tier 1 or Tier 2, then code **81479** (for unlisted molecular pathology procedure) should be used instead.

GENOMIC SEQUENCING PROCEDURES (GSPS)

Genomic sequencing procedures (GSPs) are a type of molecular pathology procedure in which multiple genes or genetic regions are tested and analyzed for medically significant issues. Unlike standard molecular pathology procedures, GSPs are used to cover a large number of related genes and sequences that may contribute to a condition. They are able to be applied to both germline and **neoplastic** (abnormal or cancerous) samples, and they are reapplied when new information is obtained. This section also includes related molecular techniques, such as the polymerase chain reaction, which are used for analysis. These procedures cover a wide variety of genetic disorders, such as those related to Ashkenazi Jew-associated disorders or hereditary cardiomyopathy.

CODING

Genomic sequencing and related procedure codes are listed by the particular class of issues that are covered by the procedure, such as fetal chromosomal aneuploidy or hearing loss. Each procedure covers a number of gene sequences that must be included in the assay. For example, code 81437 must include MAX, SDHB, SDHC, SDHD, TMEM127, and VHL in the procedure description. If an assay uses genes that are covered by multiple procedure codes, pick the most specific for the disorder being reported. Also, if only some of the gene groups are tested, but not all required gene sequences are included, report the individual codes from Tier 1 or Tier 2, or use code 81479 if the test is unlisted.

MULTIANALYTE ASSAYS WITH ALGORITHMIC ANALYSIS (MAAA) PROCEDURES

Multianalyte assays with algorithmic analysis (MAAA) procedures are specific types of laboratory and pathology procedures that combine multiple molecular and biochemical assays, patient demographics, and other clinical information into an algorithm to predict the likelihood of or risk for a disease or condition occurring in a patient. The inclusion of additional data, such as medical records and other laboratory tests, differentiates these tests from GSPs and similar multianalyte assays. MAAA procedures include the disease type, the materials analyzed and markers used, the methodology, specimen, the algorithm result, and the type of report. These codes include all of the analytic services necessary to perform the procedure, in addition to the algorithmic analysis.

CODING

MAAA procedures are listed initially by the **type of condition** that's being tested for, such as coronary artery disease or fetal congenital abnormalities. If there's a general type of condition being examined, like cancer, always confirm the specific type of condition, such as "cancer (ovarian)." If there is no additional type listed, check the **analytes being analyzed** in order to clarify the procedure.

Not all MAAA procedures are located in the "Pathology and Laboratory" section. If a procedure is not listed in that section, check **Appendix O** of the CPT book for additional codes. If the procedure is in neither location, report it using procedure code **81599**.

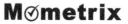

CHEMISTRY

Chemistry procedures in CPT cover the chemical analysis of body tissue or fluid specimens derived from a patient. These codes are used for the detection of specific substances that may be difficult to locate via visual inspection, such as occult blood in the feces or cholesterol in the blood. Chemistry codes are organized by the **specific analyte** being tested, such as ammonia, blood gases, or glucose, and they may be subdivided in certain cases by their **method of analysis** (such as qualitative or quantitative) or **subtype** (such as fetal chemical hemoglobin). Review the procedure notes to determine the most specific test code to report. These procedures are considered separate from a panel of tests, such as an organ- or disease-oriented panel.

HEMATOLOGY AND COAGULATION

Hematology and coagulation procedures cover laboratory and pathological examinations of a patient's blood, such as bleeding time, clotting factor tests, coagulation time, and viscosity. Codes in this section are divided by **specific procedure** being performed, although some procedures are broken down into subtypes based on the **category of the procedure**, such as clotting tests for factor II or factor VIII. These procedures may be included in certain panels or MAAA procedures. These codes only cover blood testing procedures; for procedures such as blood banking procedures or tests for agglutinins, refer to the respective sections in CPT.

IMMUNOLOGY

Immunology procedures are laboratory and pathology procedures that involve the human immune system and its various chemical and cellular components, such as antibody identification or counting the various types of white blood cells. Codes in this section are divided by the **specific procedure**, but they may be subdivided depending on the **analyte being analyzed**. For example, a total count of T cells has a different code from when a T cell count with absolute CD4 and CD8 count with ratio is performed. These procedures do not cover the analysis of specific antibodies, and they are meant to cover a comparatively general testing methodology.

QUALITATIVE IMMUNOASSAY

A qualitative immunoassay is a subset of immunology procedures involving the type and relative number of antibodies related to specific infectious diseases in the patient's blood. This also includes tests for human immunodeficiency virus (HIV). Codes in this section are divided by the **specific disease** antibodies that are being tested for, such as *Giardia lamblia* or influenza. When coding these procedures, code as specifically as possible according to the procedural notes. If multiple assays are performed for different classes of immunoglobulin, then each assay must be coded separately, despite testing for the same disease. These codes are for lengthy, multiple-step methods of antibody detection; use code 86318 for single-step and related methods.

TISSUE TYPING

Tissue typing is a form of immunological procedure that focuses on the compatibility of tissues and organs from differing sources. These procedures are typically performed prior to organ and tissue transplants in order to determine compatibility and hopefully avoid tissue rejection and similar issues. Typically, a specific tissue typing procedure is only done once, and it is recorded for all instances of transplantation involving the patient. These codes are divided by the **specific procedure**, although some have subtypes based on the specific methodology, e.g., multiple antigens versus a single antigen. The recipient of the transplant and the original donor or donors should be coded for the procedures performed.

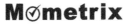

TRANSFUSIONS

Transfusion medicine is a category of laboratory and pathology procedures that covers the transfusion of blood and blood components, such as plasma or leukocytes between individual sources. This section covers a variety of procedures including antibody tests, blood typing (including paternity tests), screening for antigens, and storing of frozen blood. These codes are divided by the **specific procedure**, although some (such as blood typing) have related codes based on methodology or additional processes. These codes are for diagnostic and storage procedures; procedures such as apheresis and therapeutic phlebotomy are found elsewhere in CPT and should be coded appropriately.

MICROBIOLOGY

Microbiology procedures in CPT involve the analysis, identification, and culturing of microorganisms for the purposes of diagnosing disorders or diseases. These procedures cover a number of specialties, including **bacteriology** (the study of bacteria), **mycology** (the study of fungus), **parasitology** (the study of parasites), and **virology** (the study of viruses). Codes in this section are initially categorized by the **specific procedure**, although many codes have subcategories determined by the **methodology**, such as different analysis techniques; or the **sample source** used in the analysis or culture. These codes are meant for presumptive identification; more definitive tests require additional tests and should be coded separately. If multiple specimens are used for a test, append modifier 59 to the code. If the same test is performed multiple times on the same sample on the same day, append modifier 91 to the code.

PRIMARY SOURCE MICROBIOLOGY

Primary source microbiology procedures involve the analysis, detection, and culturing of specific infectious agents. These codes are used when the type of virus, bacteria, or other pathogen is known, either categorically (such as an adenovirus) or specifically (such as herpes simplex virus type 1). These codes are organized initially by **method of detection** and then by **general classification** of the particular pathogen. The general codes also have several subcategories based on the **specific type** of pathogen. If the specific type of infectious agent is not known, report the general methodology code as the most specific code selectable (e.g., "Not otherwise specified, each organism").

ANATOMICAL PATHOLOGY

Anatomical pathology procedures in CPT are primarily **autopsy** procedures, also known as **necropsy**, which involve the examination of a dead body by a trained physician. These codes are organized by type and level of detail: **gross, gross and microscopic, regional**, and **forensic examination**. Gross examination involves physical and visual examination of the deceased. Microscopic examination involves taking tissue samples for additional analysis. Regional autopsies cover a single bodily system or organ. Forensic autopsies are performed in the event of a criminal investigation, and they may or may not include a coroner's call of whether the death was natural, accidental, or deliberate. All codes are assumed to be performed by the physician on site; if an outside lab performs the service, use modifier 90 in conjunction with the appropriate code.

CYTOPATHOLOGY

Cytopathology procedures are pathology procedures that involve the study, analysis, and diagnosis of diseases at a cellular level, typically through the microscopic study of fragmented bodily tissue and free cells from the patient's body. Such samples can be acquired either through manual removal (such as with a wash or a needle) or through spontaneous exfoliation of cells. This also includes forensic cytopathology and DNA analysis procedures. This typically involves the removal of cells

71

through various means for study and analysis. Cytopathology procedure codes are categorized primarily by the **technique** used to analyze the samples provided, such as in situ hybridization. Gynecological cytopathology procedures are coded separately from more generalized cytopathology procedures.

GYNECOLOGICAL

This section of cytopathology procedures focuses primarily on **gynecological** procedures, or procedures involving the female reproductive system. Typically, these codes will involve acquiring samples from the cervix or vagina for study and screening. These procedures are organized primarily by the **method of screening**, such as manual screening or automated thin layer preparation, although several procedures will have related codes that cover rescreening by the physician. In addition, check the procedural notes to see if the **Bethesda system**, a system for reporting pap smear results, is used during the procedure because that will alter the code selection per the notes in CPT.

CYTOGENETIC STUDIES

Cytogenetic studies are a form of molecular pathology procedures that study the relationship between **chromosomes**, the DNA molecules that contain genetic material, and diseases or conditions. These procedures involve analysis of chromosomes via visual or molecular means, as well as procedures for storing and preserving cells for later examination. Codes in this section are organized by the **specific procedure** (for storage) or **method of analysis.** Several codes use the **number of cells counted** in order to narrow down the code selection. These codes should not be used to report procedures used as part of an MAAA procedure or as part of a molecular pathology procedure; only use these codes if the cytogenetic study is being performed on its own.

SURGICAL PATHOLOGY

GROSS AND MICROSCOPIC EXAMINATION PROCEDURES

Gross and microscopic examination procedures are surgical pathology procedures that involve the analysis of tissue specimens taken from a patient for the purposes of examination and diagnosis. Examination codes are divided into **gross only** and **gross and microscopic** examinations. Gross exams include a visual inspection of the specimen, whereas gross and microscopic exams include a detailed look at the specimen under a microscope. Procedure codes related to examination are separated into levels in CPT, with Level I representing gross examination of any tissue specimen and all of the other levels representing gross and microscopic examination of various categories of tissues. If multiple specimens of the same type are taken from a single patient, then each specimen is coded as an individual, not as a group.

PROCEDURES AND CODING

Surgical pathology covers not just gross and microscopic examination of tissue samples taken from patients; additional procedure codes are given for specialized and non-microscopic analysis and examination, such as histochemical stains, morphometric analysis, and macroscopic examination and dissection. It also covers additional related procedures, such as consultations and reports on prepared tissues. Codes in this portion of the "Surgical Pathology" section are ordered by the **specific procedure**, and they often include add-on codes for procedures that may require **multiple specimens or procedures.** Always check for parentheticals underneath each procedure description because several codes may not be reported in conjunction with others located elsewhere in CPT.

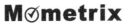

IN VIVO PROCEDURES

In vivo and miscellaneous laboratory procedures are procedures, typically noninvasive, that involve the analysis of bodily fluids or substances such as bilirubin, hemoglobin, urine, feces, sputum, and sweat in order to assess, quantify, or detect certain values or substances. These procedures are sufficiently different from other laboratory procedures, so they are placed in a separate category to differentiate them. In vivo procedures are organized based on the **specific fluid or substance** (such as bilirubin or hemoglobin) that is being analyzed, whereas miscellaneous procedures are organized based on the **procedure** and the **substance being tested for** (such as leukocytes or fat).

REPRODUCTIVE MEDICINE PROCEDURES

Reproductive medicine procedures are laboratory procedures that revolve around reproductive cells and tissues, particularly oocytes, nonimplanted embryos, and sperm. These procedures cover the analysis and identification of various reproductive cells, as well as artificial insemination and short- or long-term cryopreservation of embryos, oocytes, sperm, and reproductive tissue for later use or analysis. Procedures in this category are organized by **specific procedure** (such as cryopreservation), with additional codes related to **quantity** (in the case of fertilization or biopsy), the **specific analysis type**, or the **type of tissue being preserved** (in the case of cryopreservation). Cryopreservation and storage codes, unless otherwise specified, cover all units from a specific patient being preserved or stored.

PROPRIETARY LABORATORY ANALYSIS

Proprietary laboratory analysis procedures are special procedures that can either only be performed by a single laboratory or are owned by a specific brand or organization and licensed to multiple providing laboratories. These procedures cover a wide variety of analysis procedures, such as MAAA and GSP, but they do not technically fall into those categories due to their proprietary nature. These codes are easily identified by a "U" in the procedure code's fifth character space; there is a list of proprietary names located in **Appendix O** of the CPT handbook. Codes in this section are only reported if the type of analysis performed matches the code descriptor and falls under the proprietary name listed in **Appendix O**.

Medicine

IMMUNIZATIONS
IMMUNE GLOBULINS, SERUM, AND RECOMBINANT PRODUCTS

Immune globulins, serum, and recombinant products are a list of codes used for substances derived from blood created for the purposes of immunization. These include **immune globulins** and **serum**, which are typically derived from human blood; and **recombinant products,** which are produced via a mix of genetically altered human- and animal-sourced blood products and proteins. Codes for these products are organized by the **specific substance or disease** that the globulin, serum, or recombinant is designed to protect against, and they are meant to be used in conjunction with the appropriate administration procedure codes. For administration procedures, see codes **96365** through **96375** located later in the "Medicine" section of CPT.

ADMINISTRATION PROCEDURES

Immunization administration procedures are used when a specific vaccine or toxoid is administered to a patient to generate an immune response. These codes are used in conjunction with vaccine and toxoid product codes, and they cover the actual procedure of administering a vaccine. The codes are divided into three categories: administration with counseling (**90460**), administration via injection (**90471**), and administration via intranasal or oral route (**90473**), each with add-on codes for extra vaccines. Each additional vaccine administered is reported separately. These codes are reported separately from E/M codes if performed in conjunction with those services.

VACCINE AND TOXOID PRODUCTS

Vaccine and toxoid product codes are used to code the actual vaccines or toxoids that are administered during immunization procedures. Because these codes do not describe actual procedures, they should not be reported without the appropriate immunization procedure code (see **90460** through **90474**), nor should they be reported with modifier 51 if multiple instances of a vaccine are used. These codes are organized by the **type of disease or toxoid** that the vaccine is meant to immunize the patient from. If a patient is given a combination vaccine for multiple pathogens, then the appropriate combination vaccine code should be reported instead of the individual separate vaccine codes; e.g., do not report the hepatitis A and B vaccines separately if a combination hepatitis A and B immunization is given.

PSYCHIATRY
INTERACTIVE COMPLEXITY

Psychiatric procedures may be complicated by issues that disrupt or interfere with communication between the provider and the subject. CPT uses the term interactive complexity to refer to these issues. Typically, these factors may occur if a patient has a third party (such as a guardian, parole officer, child welfare agent, or an accompanying family member or interpreter) with them during the service. According to CPT, interactive complexity is coded when one or more of the following is demonstrated:

- Management of maladaptive communication
- Issues that interfere with a caregiver's understanding or ability to assist
- Evidence, disclosure, or discussion of an event that requires a mandated report
- Use of tools, interpreters, or translators to communicate with a patient who has difficulty speaking or understanding.

74

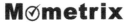

Interactive complexity is an add-on code, and it should not be reported individually or with psychotherapy for crisis.

PSYCHOTHERAPY PROCEDURES

Psychotherapy procedures are medical procedures meant to treat a patient's mental illness or behavioral issues. These typically include things like communication, helping to alleviate emotional disturbance, altering destructive or otherwise maladaptive behaviors, and encouraging positive mental development. Psychotherapy procedures are organized primarily by the **time spent** with the patient. In addition, this section includes add-on codes used in conjunction with E/M procedures performed as part of the psychotherapy procedure. If this is done, the E/M services and psychotherapy services should be separately identifiable and distinct. These codes are meant for single patients, not for family procedures.

PSYCHOTHERAPY FOR CRISIS

Psychotherapy for crisis is a psychiatric procedure meant for patients that are in a state of acute mental and psychological distress, such as a mental breakdown, severe anxiety attack, display of suicidal intent, or other extreme moments of crisis. This includes urgent assessment, treatment, and the mobilization of any resources needed to safely defuse the crisis and minimize emotional or psychological trauma. These codes are used to report the first 30 to 74 minutes of intervention involving the patient and any family members present, with an add-on code for each 30-minute block afterward. If fewer than 30 minutes are spent during the psychotherapy for crisis, CPT states that codes **90832** or **90833** (if E/M are performed) should be reported instead.

DIALYSIS

HEMODIALYSIS

Hemodialysis is a type of medical procedure that uses a machine to artificially filter wastes and excess water from the patient's blood in the place of their kidneys, typically as part of a treatment for renal disease or damage. These procedures include E/M procedures related to the disease on the day of dialysis. The procedures are separated based on whether a physician or other qualified professional performs either a single evaluation, repeated evaluation, or an access flow study during the dialysis process. CPT reveals that these codes are used for inpatient procedures and outpatient, non-end-stage renal disease (ESRD) services.

END-STAGE RENAL DISEASE (ESRD) SERVICES

End-stage renal disease (ESRD) services are dialysis procedures performed in an outpatient setting for an individual in the terminal stages of renal disease, when the kidneys are essentially nonfunctional. These services are typically used for elderly patients or individuals with chronic or sustained kidney dysfunction. These procedures include the establishment of a dialysis schedule, outpatient E/M services, and patient management, and they are reported once a month. Codes in this section are organized primarily by the **age of the patient** and then by the **number of face-to-face visits** performed by a healthcare professional per month. Alternatively, if ESRD services are provided for less than a full month, use codes **90967** through **90970** (depending on the age of the patient) with a number of units equal to the number of days.

OPHTHALMOLOGY

GENERAL OPHTHALMOLOGY SERVICES

General ophthalmology services are procedures in which an ophthalmologist provides general vision care services for a patient, which typically involve nonspecialized treatment, examinations, and other general diagnostic procedures. General services are organized primarily by whether a patient is **new** or **established**, based on E/M guidelines. After that, procedures are based on whether the services are **intermediate** or **comprehensive**. Intermediate services, as defined by CPT, are the evaluation of a new or existing condition that's been complicated by a new condition or problem. Comprehensive services, by contrast, are defined by CPT as a general examination and evaluation of the entire visual system.

SPECIAL OPHTHALMOLOGY SERVICES

Special ophthalmology services cover ophthalmology procedures that go beyond the requirements of general services or involve a special treatment or evaluation of the visual system. These services may be reported in addition to either general ophthalmology procedures or as part of a patient's E/M services. These codes include the interpretation and reporting of the results, and they may or may not include the technical component of the procedure. Procedures under this category are organized by the **specific procedure** that is being performed, such as computerized corneal topography or a visual field examination. Note any parentheticals under the procedure descriptions for alternative codes or codes that may not be used in conjunction with the selected procedure code.

OTORHINOLARYNGOLOGICAL SERVICES

Special otorhinolaryngological services are diagnostic and treatment procedures involving the ear, nose, and throat that exceed the scope of standard E/M services or outpatient consultation. These can include speech tests, vestibular function tests, evaluations of cochlear implants, and other related procedures. Codes in this section are organized by the **specific category of procedure**, such as vestibular function tests or evaluative and therapeutic services, and they are then organized by the **specific procedure type**. When coding these procedures, always check any parentheticals underneath the procedure's description for alternative codes or codes that should not be reported in conjunction with that procedure.

CARDIOVASCULAR
CORONARY THERAPEUTIC SERVICES

Coronary therapeutic service codes cover procedures meant to repair or relieve either temporary or chronic occlusion of a blood vessel. CPT describes these procedures as **percutaneous coronary intervention** procedures. These procedures include, in order of difficulty, coronary stents, percutaneous transluminal coronary angioplasties, and atherectomies, and they are performed on major coronary arteries, coronary artery branches, and CABG. Procedures in this section are organized by the **type of procedure** being performed, and they are accompanied by add-on codes indicating additional coronary branches or arteries that the procedures are performed on.

ECHOCARDIOGRAPHY

Echocardiography is a procedure in which images of the heart or great vessels are obtained via ultrasound scanning equipment, typically with real-time imaging, documentation of Doppler signals, or both. These procedures may be performed at rest, as part of a cardiovascular stress test, or both. These codes are organized by the chosen **method of approach** (either transthoracic or transesophageal), then by the **types of imaging** that are used during the scan (such as a spectral Doppler echocardiography), and finally by whether the procedure is part of a **stress test**. Procedures in this section include the interpretation and documentation of the scan's results.

CARDIAC CATHETERIZATION

Cardiac catheterization procedures are a type of diagnostic procedure involving the insertion and positioning of a **catheter** (a long, thin tube) for the purposes of analyzing blood flow, intracardiac and intravascular pressure, blood oxygen saturation, and other information. These procedures can

76

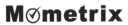

be performed on both sides or on either side of the heart (left or right), and they are typically performed on patients with congenital heart disease or other heart-related issues. These procedures are organized based on the **procedure** being performed (left, right, or combined left and right heart catheterization or angiography), although many codes (**93455** through **93461**) are additional codes for coronary angiography (code **93454**).

PULMONARY AND ALLERGY
PULMONARY DIAGNOSTIC TESTING AND THERAPY

Pulmonary diagnostic testing and therapy covers procedures that involve diagnostic analysis and treatment of the lungs and pulmonary system, including analysis of air flow, lung volume, pulmonary function, and other data; as well as inhalation treatments with aerosolized medication. These procedures are organized by the **specific procedure**, and they include all of the necessary laboratory procedures and interpretation of results by a physician. Always check the parentheticals under each procedure description for alternative codes and for codes that may not be reported in conjunction with the specific procedure. These procedures may be performed in conjunction with E/M procedures; if so, then report the appropriate code in conjunction with the codes in this section.

ALLERGEN IMMUNOTHERAPY PROCEDURES

Allergen immunotherapy is a type of medical procedure in which a patient is slowly desensitized to environmental allergens in order to strengthen the patient's immune system and reduce harmful responses. For these procedures, the proper code can be determined if the procedure notes discuss whether the immunotherapy is only administered (in the case of codes **95115** and **95117**), if the immunotherapy is provided and administered (in the case of codes **95120** through **95134**), or if the immunotherapy is only prepared and not administered to the patient (in the case of codes **95144** through **95170**). In addition, the specific type of immunotherapy, such as insect venom, should be taken into account. In all cases, care should be taken to review the provided procedural notes.

NEUROLOGY AND CENTRAL NERVOUS SYSTEM
SLEEP MEDICINE TESTING

Sleep medicine covers procedures used to evaluate pediatric and adult patients for issues involving or occurring during the sleep cycle, such as sleep apnea or insomnia. These services are primarily diagnostic, and they include recording, interpreting, and reporting data as part of the procedure. Codes in this section are organized primarily by the **procedure performed**, and they are further subdivided by **any additional analysis performed** as a part of the study, e.g., respiratory analysis during a sleep study, or by the **age of the participant** in certain cases. If a study has fewer than 6 hours recorded during the procedure, append modifier 52 to the appropriate code.

CENTRAL NERVOUS SYSTEM ASSESSMENTS

Central nervous system assessments are medical tests meant to examine a patient's sensory neurons and cognitive functions to see if the nervous system is somehow impaired or underdeveloped. These assessments include memory and language, visual and auditory, and abstract reasoning skills testing. Procedures in this section are divided by the **specific type of assessment**, such as aphasia or neurobehavioral status examination, and they are further subdivided by the **time taken** during the procedure. For these codes, each given block of time (such as 1 hour or 30 minutes) counts as a single unit for the purposes of coding. For example, if an aphasia assessment takes 2 hours, the proper code to report would be 96105 × 2.

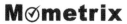

HYDRATION PROCEDURES

Hydration procedures involve the intravenous injection of fluids, typically a mix of saline, dextrose, electrolytes, and other fluids. This can be performed to help a patient suffering from dehydration or nutrient deficiency recover quickly, or it can be performed with an included mixture of therapeutic or diagnostic medicine as part of a treatment program. These procedures are organized by the **time spent** during the procedure, typically in 1-hour blocks after the initial introduction. It should be noted that, in the case of hydration without drug infusion, the minimum time for infusion is 30 minutes. Infusions shorter than this should not be reported. For shorter times involving the introduction of drugs or other therapeutic substances, see code **96372** for injections.

CHEMOTHERAPY PROCEDURES

Chemotherapy is a procedure in which highly complex **antineoplastic** (anticancer) drugs or other biological agents are administered to a patient for the purposes of treatment, typically for the purposes of destroying malignant lesions or tumors. Chemotherapy can be introduced either intravenously, via intramuscular injection directly into the lesion or lesions, or via various intra-arterial means. These procedures are organized by the **method of introduction** (intravenous or intra-arterial) and then either by the **number of lesions** (for intralesional) or the **length of infusion**, with add-on codes for time intervals greater than 30 minutes. The codes for the specific drugs should be coded separately because these codes only cover the actual administration of the treatment.

PHOTODYNAMIC THERAPY

Photodynamic therapy is a type of dermatological procedure used to treat cancerous and noncancerous lesions of the skin and related tissue via photosensitive drugs. After the drugs are applied, high-intensity light is used to activate the drugs, which then destroy the cells of any tissue that the drugs are applied to. The main procedures are organized by whether the treatment is **performed by a physician** or not. In addition, the section includes add-on codes for photodynamic therapy used for treating internal lesions, such as in the lungs or gastrointestinal system. These add-on codes are differentiated by the **duration of treatment**, and they should be reported in addition to the appropriate bronchoscopy or endoscopy codes.

SPECIAL DERMATOLOGICAL PROCEDURES

Special dermatological procedures are miscellaneous procedures involving diagnostic analysis and treatment of skin issues. These include procedures such as ultraviolet light therapy, laser treatment of psoriasis, and reflectance confocal microscopy, as well as otherwise unlisted dermatological procedures. Because these procedures do not fit in with other procedural categories, they are filed under this category. Codes in this category are organized by **type of procedure**. Codes for reflectance confocal microscopy have a number of additional codes that are used to better report this particular procedure, in addition to add-on codes for each additional lesion that the particular procedure is performed on.

PHYSICAL MEDICINE AND REHABILITATION

Physical medicine and rehabilitation procedures cover a specific type of medical evaluation used for physical therapy, occupational therapy, and athletic training evaluations. Similar to standard E/M procedures, physical medicine and rehabilitation codes typically include an assessment that contains medical history, an examination of systems, and clinical decision making, and they list a typical amount of time spent on face-to-face contact with the providing physician. However, there are differences: Physical therapy requires a clinical presentation of changing characteristics, while occupational therapy assesses issues that may impede work. Codes in this section are first separated into the **type of evaluation** and then by the **level of complexity**, e.g., low, medium, or high. Each procedure requires that all components must be included in order to be accurately coded, regardless of patient status.

MODALITIES

Modalities, as referred to in this section of CPT, refer to a variety of therapeutic methods that attempt to produce positive changes in a patient's condition. These procedures are typically noninvasive, and they cover things such as heat and cold packs, electrostimulation, or exposure to infrared or ultraviolet light. Modalities are divided into **supervised** procedures, which do not require direct contact with the patient; and **constant attendance**, which requires the presence of a provider. These procedures are listed by the **specific method** used. In the case of modalities requiring constant attendance, codes are listed in units of 15 minutes. For example, a 30-minute contrast bath would be coded as 97034 twice.

THERAPEUTIC PROCEDURES

Therapeutic procedures cover a wide variety of physical, social, and psychological services aimed at improving a patient's physical, cognitive, or social functionality. In addition to physical exercises and manipulation, therapeutic procedures also include forms of training, such as wheelchair use and community integration training, that allows the patient to work or interact with others. These procedures require direct contact between the patient and the provider. Procedures in this category are grouped by the **specific procedure**, and they are often listed in units of time (typically in blocks of 15 minutes). For example, 1 hour of gait training would be coded as four instances of code 97116.

ACUPUNCTURE

Acupuncture procedures are a form of alternative medicine that involves the insertion of needles into key positions on the body for relief of certain symptoms. The insertion of the needles may also be accompanied by a mild electrical stimulation via a current run through the needles. Acupuncture services are reported in units of 15 minutes, and they are organized depending on whether the procedure does or does not use **electrical stimulation** through the needles. When reporting, the code for an initial procedure is only used once per day; multiple instances of treatment should be counted via add-on codes.

OSTEOPATHIC AND CHIROPRACTIC MANIPULATION PROCEDURES

Osteopathic and chiropractic procedures are a form of alternative medicine involving the manipulation of body parts for relief of pain, stiffness, and other certain symptoms. Osteopathic manipulation treatment involves the manipulation of muscles and bones, whereas chiropractic manipulation treatment involves the manipulation of the spinal column. These procedures are organized by the **number of bodily regions** that are manipulated by the provider, and they typically include a pre-manipulation assessment of the patient. A list of bodily regions used for osteopathic manipulation treatment and chiropractic manipulation treatment procedures are provided in the relevant sections. If the provider performs E/M services on the patient, code them separately from the actual osteopathic and chiropractic procedures.

PATIENT EDUCATION AND TRAINING

Education and training procedures cover educational and instruction services prescribed and provided by a qualified health professional to a nonqualified individual, such as the patient, patient's guardian, or caregiver for the purpose of treating an established illness or minimizing or delaying further issues. These procedures are different from the counseling and education provided as part of an E/M service because they typically involve education beyond what such a service

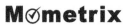

would entail. Procedures of this type are organized by the **number of individual patients or caregivers** that undergo education, and they are coded in blocks of 30 minutes. These services are meant for individuals; for group training, see code **99078**.

NON-FACE-TO-FACE SERVICES

Non-face-to-face services are a type of patient assessment, separate from E/M, that takes place over a long distance between a qualified healthcare professional and a patient or their guardian or caregiver. These types of services can be performed either over the telephone or via online communications, the latter of which must include recording and permanent storage of the encounter. Codes related to these procedures are organized by the **method of communication**, either telephone or online. Codes for telephone communications are determined by the total amount of time spent in medical discussion. The codes for telephone communication are not reported if the communication leads to a face-to-face encounter within 24 hours or the nearest available urgent appointment.

MODERATE SEDATION

ACTIVITIES INVOLVED IN MODERATE SEDATION SERVICES

Moderate sedation, also known as **conscious sedation**, is a form of anesthesia in which a patient remains conscious enough to respond to verbal or tactile commands, while able to breathe on their own without assistance. These sorts of procedures differ from MAC in that the physicians themselves perform the sedation instead of a separate anesthesiologist. Moderate sedation services include **preservice**, **intraservice**, and **postservice** work. Preservice includes assessment of the patient's history, allergies, and vital signs before sedation. Intraservice work begins with the actual administration of the sedation, and it is used to determine the proper CPT code to be used. Finally, postservice work includes postsedation assessments and readiness for discharge.

PROCEDURES AND CODING

Moderate sedation procedures are identified by the lack of an anesthesiologist or certified registered nurse anesthesiologist performing the actual procedure; instead, the physicians themselves provide the sedation service. These codes are primarily organized by whether an **independent trained observer** is present to assist in monitoring the patient's level of consciousness and physical status. Codes are further separated by the **age of the patient**, with 5 years old being the dividing line. Codes indicate the amount of intraservice time in blocks of 15 minutes. For example, if a 6-year-old patient undergoes moderate sedation with observation for 45 minutes, then the proper codes to report would be 99152 once and 99153 twice.

International Classification of Diseases, 10th Revision, Clinical Modification (ICD-10-CM)

STRUCTURE OF (ICD-10-CM) CODES

Unlike CPT, ICD-10-CM codes consist of a set of up to seven characters and a decimal point that indicate the position of the diagnosis in ICD-10-CM and various other pieces of relevant information. Generally speaking, ICD-10-CM codes are structured as follows:

- Each code begins with a **letter**, indicating the general category of the code in the tabular list. For example, L is for a skin condition.
- After the letter are **two numbers**, which further narrow the code's position in the listing and general type of condition. For example, L02 is for a cutaneous abscess.
- The first three characters are followed by a **decimal** to separate the general category from the specifics.
- The **fourth character** is used to narrow the diagnosis further. For example, L02.2 is for a cutaneous abscess of the trunk.
- The **fifth and sixth characters** provide the most specific diagnosis. For example, L02.211 is for a cutaneous abscess of the abdominal wall.
- A **seventh character** is typically used for additional information, such as the time of the encounter.
- If there are missing characters between the rest of the code and the seventh character, a **placeholder "X"** is used in place of the missing characters, e.g., M48.40**X**A.

ICD-10-CM TABULAR LIST

The color-coded tabular list makes up the bulk of the ICD-10-CM coding book. The tabular list contains all of the diagnosis codes that have been officially added to ICD-10-CM, and it is arranged into sections based on general anatomical category or similar commonalities. The tabular list contains the following sections:

- **A through B**: Infectious and parasitic diseases
- **C through D49**: Neoplasms (e.g., cancer)
- **D50 through D89**: Blood, blood-forming organs, and certain immune disorders
- **E:** Endocrine, nutritional, and metabolic diseases
- **F:** Mental, behavioral, and neurodevelopmental disorders
- **G:** Nervous system
- H (H00 through H59): Eye and adnexa
- **H (H60 through H95)**: Ear and mastoid process
- **I:** Circulatory system
- **J:** Respiratory system
- **K:** Digestive system
- **L:** Skin and subcutaneous tissue
- **M:** Musculoskeletal system and connective tissue
- **N:** Genitourinary system (male and female)
- **O:** Pregnancy, childbirth, and the **puerperium** (six weeks post childbirth)

- **P:** Conditions originating in the **perinatal** (immediately before and after birth) period
- **Q:** Congenital malformations, deformations, and chromosomal abnormalities
- **R:** Symptoms, signs, and abnormal findings
- **S through T:** Injury and poisoning
- **V through Y:** Factors influencing health status and contact with health services.

SELECTING THE CORRECT ICD-10-CM DIAGNOSIS CODE

The ICD-10-CM coding book is used to code the condition that the patient is diagnosed with, based on the procedural notes provided. Although some diagnoses, such as cancer, injury, or poison, require additional or alternative steps, the vast majority of diagnosis code selection involves the following steps:

1. **Look up the diagnosis in the index.** The index lists all of the diagnoses provided in ICD-10-CM in alphabetical order by the name of the condition, with indented subcategories listed underneath for more specific diagnoses. For example, a diagnosis of type 2 diabetes with polyneuropathy would be listed under **"Diabetes,"** followed by **"type 2, with,"** and then **"polyneuropathy."**
2. **Follow the code listed in the index to the proper code in the tabular list.** Once the condition is found in the index, follow the given code to the location in the tabular list. **Do not just use the code given in the index**; some codes are incomplete or may require additional characters.
3. **Report the codes in the proper sequence.** When coding diagnoses, the proper sequence is the order in which the conditions are mentioned in the procedural notes unless stated otherwise in ICD-10-CM.

CODING NEOPLASM DIAGNOSES USING ICD-10-CM

Unlike other conditions, neoplasms (an abnormal cell growth, such as a tumor) have a separate section within the ICD-10-CM book. Neoplasms are listed in a special table based on their anatomical location, with subcategories for more precise locations. For example, a neoplasm in the transverse colon would be found under **"intestine,"** then **"large, colon,"** and **"transverse."** ICD-10-CM also divides neoplasm codes by their behavior, which falls into six categories:

1. **Malignant primary**, where a cancer has spread from
2. **Malignant secondary**, where a cancer has spread to
3. **Carcinoma in situ**, for a malignant mass isolated to a single place
4. **Benign**, for noncancerous neoplasms
5. **Uncertain behavior**, for neoplasms whose behavior has not yet been identified
6. **Unspecified behavior**, for neoplasms whose behavior is not outlined in the procedural notes.

A majority of neoplasm codes will be found in sections C and D of the tabular list. Always check the code in the tabular list after locating it in the index.

CODING INJURY DIAGNOSES USING ICD-10-CM

Injuries, much like neoplasms and drugs, are given their own separate section in the ICD-10-CM index. Injuries are listed alphabetically by the source of the injury, with indented subcategories for more precise descriptions. For example, if a patient's injury was caused when they were hit by a thrown baseball during a game they were participating in, the indexed location would be struck, then object, thrown, in sports, ball, and finally baseball. Like disease codes, it is always considered

82

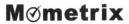

best practice to go to the code location in the tabular list to verify before reporting because some codes may require an additional character or characters that are not listed in the index.

CODING DRUG-RELATED DIAGNOSES USING ICD-10-CM

Like neoplasms and injuries, diagnoses involving drugs have a special section in the ICD-10-CM index. The table of drugs and chemicals provides an alphabetical list for all common drugs and chemicals found in medical diagnoses, with subcategories for more precise definitions. For example, if a patient was exposed to ammonia fumes from a household cleaner, it would be listed under **"ammonia (fumes) (gas) (vapor),"** then **"liquid (household)"**. The table also provides six categories for how the substance was used, as follows:

- **Poisoning, accidental**, when a patient unintentionally consumed toxic amounts of a substance
- **Poisoning, intentional, self-harm**, when a patient intentionally consumed toxic amounts of a substance
- **Poisoning, assault**, when a patient was exposed to toxic amounts of a substance by another individual
- **Poisoning, undetermined**, for when the cause of the patient's poisoning is unclear or unlisted
- **Adverse effect**, when a patient has a poor response (such as an allergic response) to a drug or substance
- **Underdosing**, when a patient is given an insufficient amount of a drug.

Most codes will be found in the "T" section of ICD-10-CM. Always check the code in the tabular list before reporting it.

Healthcare Common Procedure Coding System (HCPCS) Level II

MODIFIERS

CODING SYSTEM (HCPCS) MODIFIERS

Modifiers are alphabetic, numeric, or alphanumeric codes that are added to the end of CPT and HCPCS Level II codes to report specific modifications or alterations to the service or medical equipment without altering the code itself. These modifiers are used to more accurately report the procedure that the code describes for the purposes of billing and reimbursement of providers and suppliers.

When multiple modifiers may be appended to a single code, they must be listed in a specific way in order to be accurate. **Functional** modifiers, which alter the actual pricing of a procedure, are reported first in sequence. **Informational** modifiers, which clarify certain aspects of a procedure, such as laterality or anatomical position, are reported after functional modifiers. For example, if a bilateral procedure (modifier 50, an informational modifier) is discontinued (modifier 53, a functional modifier), then the ordering of the codes would be (CPT procedure code)-53-50.

COMMON HCPCS MODIFIERS USED WITH CPT CODES

Although HCPCS provides a wide variety of modifiers to cover different situations, not every modifier will be used regularly while coding procedures. Some modifiers are more common than others, and it pays to keep them in mind. These modifiers include the following:

22	Increased procedural service, meaning that the service was greater than what is typically required
26	Indicates the professional component, meaning that the individual who performs the procedure uses equipment or staff provided by a separate facility
51	Multiple procedures performed during a single session
52	Reduced services, meaning the service was less than what is typically required
53	Discontinued procedure, meaning the service was stopped due to circumstances
59	Distinct services, to indicate a procedure that is distinctly separate from other procedures performed in the same session
76	Repeat service by the same physician or other qualified healthcare professional

HCPCS MODIFIERS FOR ANATOMIC POSITIONING WITH CPT CODES

Certain HCPCS modifiers are used to indicate where on the body a procedure is performed. Generally speaking, some codes are required to determine the **laterality** of a procedure, such as the following:

50	Bilateral (both sides) procedure
LT	A procedure done on the left side
RT	A procedure done on the right side

84

Other codes are used to define a **specific location**, typically used for the eyelids, fingers, toes, and arteries, such as the following:

- **E1 and E2**: Upper and lower left side of the eyelid
- **E3 and E4**: Upper and lower right side of the eyelid
- **FA, F1, F2, F3, and F4**: Thumb through fifth digit, left hand
- **F5, F6, F7, F8, and F9**: Thumb through fifth digit, right hand
- **TA, T1, T2, T3, and T4**: Great toe through fifth digit, left foot
- **T5, T6, T7, T8, and T9**: Great toe through fifth digit, right foot
- **LC, LD, and LM**: The left circumflex, left anterior descending, and left main coronary arteries
- **RC and RI**: The right coronary and ramus intermedius coronary artery.

Take note in the code descriptions of which of these modifiers are not used with that particular code.

HCPCS MODIFIERS FOR PAYABLE SERVICES WITHIN A GLOBAL PACKAGE

Certain HCPCS modifiers are used during surgeries that are considered to be within what CPT refers to as a global package. A global package, as defined by CPT, consists of all procedures that occur before, during, and after (within a certain period of time) a specific surgical procedure, including any complications or postsurgical pain management. The modifiers commonly used for these include the following:

24	Unrelated E/M services by the same physician during the postoperative period
25	Significant, separate E/M service by the same physician on the same day as the procedure
57	The decision for surgery is made, such as in an emergency situation
58	Staged (i.e., done in stages over time) procedures by the same physician during the postoperative period
78	Unplanned return to the operating room by the same physician following the initial or a related procedure during the postoperative period
79	Unrelated procedure or service provided by the same physician during the postoperative period

SUPPLIES
GENERAL RULES FOR CODING

HCPCS supply codes are five-character alphanumeric codes used when coding medical supplies and services provided via Medicare and other similar insurance providers. HCPCS codes are differentiated from CPT codes in that they begin with an alphabetic character as opposed to a number, although they share a similar reporting method. Whenever a specific drug or device is mentioned in a procedure code and is noted as being provided to a patient with Medicare, an HCPCS code should be used. When coding from HCPCS, first check the alphabetical index in order to locate the appropriate code, and then check in the appropriate section to confirm the code selection before adding it.

LOCATIONS AND CATEGORIZATIONS OF SUPPLY CODES

Medical supply codes, meaning physical, nondrug equipment and supplies used in the treating of patients, are spread throughout HCPCS in a variety of categories. Generally speaking, medical supplies are divided into the following locations:

- **A4206 through A8004**: Medical and surgical supplies, such as gauze, scalpels, and drainage tubes
- **B4034 through B9999:** Enteral and parenteral therapy supplies
- **C1713 through C9899**: Outpatient prospective payment system, including implantable equipment such as pacemakers
- **E0100 through E8002:** Durable medical equipment, such as wheelchairs or commode chairs
- **K0001 through K0900**: Temporary durable medical equipment codes
- **L5000 through L9900**: Prosthetics and implants, such as extremity replacements and hernia mesh.

Codes in these sections are organized alphabetically by the **general category** of equipment, followed by the **specific type of equipment.**

MEDICATIONS

CODING OF DRUGS AND MEDICATIONS

The majority of drugs and medications are listed in section "J" of the HCPCS Level II codebook. These codes cover drugs that are administered via methods other than oral consumption, such as injection or inhalation, and they include a wide variety of pharmaceuticals. Certain other drugs, such as chemotherapy medications and oral medicines, can be found in section "Q" of HCPCS. Codes in section "J" are organized initially by the **method of administration** (such as injection), alphabetically by the **name of the drug**, and then by dosage. Some drugs will have additional, alternative names listed underneath the description (e.g., the drug baclofen may also be referred to as Gablofen or Lioresal). Always read the procedure notes to confirm the name of the drug that is administered.

EFFECTIVELY CODING DRUGS AND BIOLOGICALS USING APPENDIX A

HCPCS provides a table of drugs and biological agents, generic and brand name, in **Appendix A** of the HCPCS book. In addition to an alphabetical list, the index includes the standard unit of measurement, the route of application, and the appropriate code to be used for each drug. The unit of measurement determines how many times the code is used based on the amount given. For example, if a patient is given 50 mg of acetaminophen, that would be five units because acetaminophen is described in doses of 10 mg. This table should be used in tandem with the index in order to accurately report drugs listed in the procedure notes provided.

PROFESSIONAL SERVICES

Service codes, meaning services that are performed on or with a patient for the purposes of treatment or investigation, are spread throughout HCPCS in a variety of categories. Generally speaking, professional services are divided into the following locations:

- **A0021 through A0999**: Transportation services, including ambulances
- **A9150 through A9999**: Administrative, investigational, and miscellaneous diagnostic services
- **G0008 through G9987**: Professional services and procedures such as oncology
- **H0001 through H2037**: Alcohol and drug abuse treatment

- **L0112 through L4631**: Orthotic procedures and services
- **M0075 through M1144**: Medical services not otherwise classified
- **P2028 through P9615**: Pathology and laboratory services
- **R0070 through R0076**: Diagnostic radiology services
- V2020 through V2799: Vision services
- **V5008 through V5364**: Hearing services.

Codes of these types are organized by the **specific services** that are involved.

Coding Guidelines

ICD-10-CM OFFICIAL GUIDELINES

COMMON CODING CONVENTIONS

The ICD-10-CM guidebook uses a variety of terms, abbreviations, and symbols in order to quickly and accurately provide information with minimal space requirements. Knowledge of these conventions is necessary in order to quickly code diagnoses. Common coding conventions used by the ICD-10-CM guidebook include items from the following table:

Item		Use
-	Hyphen	Used in the index to indicate that there are additional characters associated with the code.
NEC	Not elsewhere classified	This means there isn't a code for that specific condition.
NOS	Not otherwise specified	Shorthand for "unspecified."
[ ]	Brackets	Used for manifestation codes in the index and synonyms or explanatory phrases in the tabular list.
( )	Parentheses	Enclose supplementary words or terms used for the condition.
INCLUDES		The conditions listed after this are covered by this code.
EXCLUDES1		The conditions listed after this are not coded with this code.
EXCLUDES2		The conditions listed after this are not part of the condition, but the patient may have both conditions at the same time.
Code First		Indicates a code or type of code that should be sequenced before this code.

GENERAL GUIDELINES

There are general guidelines when coding using ICD-10-CM that should always be followed in order to accurately and correctly report diagnoses. As a general rule, the following general guidelines should be followed when reporting ICD-10-CM codes:

- **Only code-confirmed conditions or diseases.** If a condition is only suspected or possible but not confirmed, then it should not be coded.
- **Code to the highest level of specificity.** Do not simply select a general code if a more focused and precise code is otherwise available.
- **Codes provided should support the medical necessity of treatment.** The codes provided must accurately reflect the available facts. In other words, no speculation is allowed.
- Each unique code should be only reported once per encounter.
- Unless otherwise specified, code the diagnoses in the order listed on the procedural notes.

CODING SIGNS AND SYMPTOMS

Signs and symptoms refer to non-diagnosis codes used for identifying individual, unrelated conditions, such as sneezing or fever. Such issues may or may not be associated with other

88

conditions listed in the procedural notes. ICD-10-CM has a few guidelines related to this particular case of coding:

- If signs and symptoms **are present, but a definitive diagnosis has not been confirmed**, then any listed signs and symptoms should be coded individually using the appropriate codes found in the tabular index.
- If the signs and symptoms are an integral part of or are routinely associated with the confirmed diagnosis, then they are not separately coded.
- If the signs and symptoms **are not routinely associated with the confirmed diagnosis**, then they should be coded individually with the appropriate codes.

CODING SEQUELA

Sequela is a medical term used for leftover or residual conditions that occur after an illness or injury has been handled, typically caused by the initial problem. Examples of sequelae include things like chronic arthritis after fracturing a wrist, severe scarring after a burn, or aphasia after a brain hemorrhage. Sequelae may occur immediately following the condition, or they may occur months or even years later; there is no time limit for sequelae to occur. When a sequela is diagnosed in a patient, the **sequela condition** is coded first, followed by the appropriate **sequela (of) code.** For example, if a patient develops an intellectual disability due to poliomyelitis, the codes sequenced should be F79 (unspecified intellectual disability), followed by B91 (sequela of poliomyelitis). The exception to this is if the code identifies the condition as following another condition, such as I69.120 (aphasia following nontraumatic intracerebral hemorrhage).

CODING HIV

The ICD-10-CM guidelines have a list of guidelines regarding how to appropriately code patients that have human immunodeficiency virus (HIV) and how it interacts with related conditions, as outlined below:

- Only code confirmed cases of HIV. In addition, the code for HIV (B20) should be included in all future cases of a patient with confirmed HIV.
- If a patient's condition is **related to HIV**, then the first diagnosis should be HIV (code B20), followed by the related conditions.
- If an HIV-positive patient is admitted for an **unrelated condition**, code the unrelated condition first, and then code the HIV.
- If a patient has **inconclusive or asymptomatic HIV status**, code B20 first if the condition is HIV related, or code the condition first followed by code Z21 if the condition isn't HIV related.

SEQUENCING NEOPLASM CODES

Neoplasm codes are mostly located in their specific section of the index in ICD-10-CM, and they have several guidelines for the proper sequencing of multiple types of codes. Common sequencing codes are as follows:

- When coding treatment of a **primary malignancy**, code the primary site first and then any secondary metastasized sites.
- When coding treatment of **secondary malignancy**, code the metastatic sites first and then the primary site.
- If the patient is undergoing treatment for a **non-anemia-related complication** related to a neoplasm, code the complication first and then the neoplasm.

- If a patient is being treated for **anemia related to a neoplasm**, code the neoplasm first and then code D63.0 (anemia in neoplastic disease).
- If a patient is being seen for a **pathological fracture due to a neoplasm**, code the focus of the treatment first.
- If a primary malignancy has been excised but **further treatment** is being performed, code the primary malignancy until treatment is completed. Afterward, if there is no evidence of malignancy at that site, use the appropriate code from category Z85.

Coding Diabetes

ICD-10-CM has several guidelines for properly coding diabetes mellitus, one of the most common endocrine diseases. Common guidelines are as follows:

- If the type of diabetes mellitus is not specified in the procedure notes or the medical record, code the condition as type 2 diabetes mellitus (E11).
- If the type of diabetes mellitus is not specified and the procedure notes include the use of insulin, code type 2 diabetes mellitus and include an additional code from category Z79 to identify long-term use of insulin or hypoglycemic drugs.
- If the type of diabetes is gestational diabetes caused by pregnancy, assign a code from subcategory O24.4 instead of the standard diabetes code.

Coding Hypertensive Heart Disease and Chronic Kidney Disease

Hypertensive heart disease and chronic kidney disease are two conditions that are commonly **comorbid** (meaning they occur simultaneously) in a patient, enough that the situation has dedicated guidelines when it is coded in ICD-10-CM. Unless the procedural notes state that the two conditions are unrelated, the condition should be sequenced as follows:

1. Code from combination category **I13** for hypertension with heart and kidney involvement.
2. If heart failure is present, use the appropriate code from category **I50.**
3. Code from category **N18** to identify the stage of chronic kidney disease.
4. If the patient is suffering from acute renal failure as well, code the level of renal failure last in the sequence.

Coding External Causes of Morbidity

External causes of morbidity is the term that ICD-10-CM uses to indicate an injury or condition that was caused by outside forces, such as car accidents, falls, acts of God, and so on. These codes can be used to elaborate on how a condition was caused; the intent behind it (accidental, intentional, or otherwise); where the event that caused the condition occurred; as well as the patient's status, whether military, civilian, etc.

External-cause codes are not sequenced first, and they are only used in conjunction with codes from other ranges if an external cause is mentioned. Typically, they'll be used with injuries or poisonings. When coding, use as many external cause codes as necessary to fully represent the condition as it is explained in the procedural notes.

Coding Patient Histories

Patient histories are coded using codes from section "Z" in the tabular list, covering code categories **Z80** through **Z87, Z91.4, Z91.5, Z91.81, Z91.82,** and **Z92.** History codes are divided into two different types: **personal** and **family.** Personal history codes are used when a procedure mentions a patient's past medical condition that may be relevant to the current condition or requires monitoring, and they are used in conjunction with follow-up codes. Family history codes are used when the procedural notes mention that a patient has familial history that may put them at risk for certain conditions, and they are used in conjunction with screening codes to establish medical necessity. Either type is acceptable on a medical record for the reason for the visit.

SCREENING CODES

Screening codes are used for encounters that focus on testing for signs and precursors of diseases in seemingly healthy individuals, typically for the purposes of early detection and treatment of a condition. Screening codes are listed in section "Z" of the tabular list in sections "**Z11**" through "**Z13**" and "**Z36**," and they are used to indicate that a screening has been planned. If the purpose of the encounter is specifically for the screening exam, then the screening code is sequenced first. If a condition is discovered during the screening, the code for the condition should be sequenced separately after the screening code.

CPT

COMMON CONVENTIONS FOR CODES

The CPT guidebook uses a variety of symbols and formatting in order to present information in a way that can be easily referenced and understood by the reader. Knowledge of these conventions helps the reader to quickly understand codes at a glance and how they are referenced. Important conventions for coding are listed below:

- **Indentation**: A code description that is indented is used to indicate a modification of the non-indented code listed above it. For example, the code 21462, "with interdental fixation," is indented underneath code 21461, "open treatment of mandibular fracture; without interdental fixation." Therefore, the appropriate way to read code 21462 is "open treatment of mandibular fracture; with interdental fixation."
- **+:** The "plus" sign indicates that the code is an **add-on code**, meaning that it adds on to an existing code. Add-on codes cannot be reported on their own.
- **⊘**: The "no" symbol indicates that the code is exempted from modifier 51.
- **Red text**: Bright red text indicates that the code in question has been moved to another location in the CPT guidebook. Read the text to see where the code has been moved to.

CRITERIA USED FOR CODE CATEGORIES

CPT codes are defined by the American Medical Association and are separated into three categories based on the frequency of clinical use, clearance by the appropriate oversight bodies, and levels of monetary value. CPT code categories are listed below:

- **Category I**: This category is used for procedures cleared or approved by the FDA that are frequently performed and documented. These codes make up the bulk of CPT's codes and cover E/M, anesthesia, surgery, radiology, pathology, and laboratory and medicine. These codes have five digits.
- **Category II:** This category is used for reporting procedures usually included in E/M or clinical services but are not associated with the typical fees or values. These codes are made up of four numbers followed by the letter F.
- **Category III:** This category covers codes used for temporary or experimental procedures or services. Codes in this category are made up of four numbers followed by the letter T.

REPORTING OF UNLISTED PROCEDURES

Despite its regular updates, the CPT codebook does not list every single procedure that may be performed by a physician or other qualified healthcare provider. In the event that a procedure is performed that is currently unlisted by CPT, each section of CPT has a designated code, typically ending in 99, that is used to report unlisted procedures or services. For example, an unlisted procedure involving the lacrimal system would use code 68899. These codes should only be used if a more appropriate code is not available or if CPT references the unlisted procedure code's use in a parenthetical note.

PARENTHETICALS

Parentheticals, also known as parenthetical notes, refer to additional information used to supplement a procedural code or to aid in accurately coding procedures in CPT. Parentheticals are so named for the use of parentheses to bracket either end of the note. Parentheticals are used in several different ways, including presenting additional codes that may be involved in a procedure, listing codes that should or should not be reported in conjunction with a particular code, guiding the reader to related procedures, and other advisory notes. When in doubt on a procedure, always check for any parenthetical notes that may be included.

HCPCS

COMMON SYMBOLS AND CONVENTIONS

HCPCS uses symbols and text conventions to provide necessary information to code Medicare procedures without taking up excess space. Knowledge of these symbols and conventions will allow a coder to quickly and accurately code procedures in HCPCS. Commonly used conventions are listed below:

- **Letter in a block**: A letter in a blue block is used to identify circumstances affecting payment: **C** means carrier judgment, **D** means that special coverage instructions apply, **I** means not payable by Medicare, **M** means noncovered by Medicare, and **S** means noncovered by Medicare statute.
- **Colored text**: Colored text is used for indicators: **Green** is used for ambulatory surgical center (ASC) indicators, **red** is used for ambulatory payment calculator indicators, and **purple** indicates an ASC-approved procedure.
- **Blue text**: Blue text is used for alerts, such as "Service not separately priced by Part B."
- **DME**: This text in a purple box means that the procedure is paid under a durable medical equipment fee schedule.
- **MIPS**: This text in a light-blue box indicates that the code is covered under the merit-based incentive payment system (MIPS).

TYPES OF CODES

HCPCS covers a variety of codes that are classified as Level II codes, comparable to CPT's Level I codes. The HCPCS is used to efficiently code and process claims for products and services across a wide variety of fields and states, including a wide variety of manufacturers. Most of the codes in HCPCS can be divided into the three categories listed below:

- **Permanent national codes**: Permanent national codes are maintained by the Centers for Medicare and Medicare Services (CMS) and are used by all public and private health insurers. These codes make up the bulk of the HCPCS codes provided.
- **Miscellaneous codes:** These codes are used when a supplier or provider submits a bill for a service or item that currently lacks an appropriate permanent national code. These codes are typically used for items or services that are rarely used.
- **Temporary national codes**: Temporary national codes are used to meet the operational needs of a particular insurer within a short time frame. Unlike miscellaneous codes, temporary national codes may be made into permanent codes.

Compliance and Regulatory

MEDICARE
MEDICARE PART A

Medicare Part A is part of the United States government's insurance plan that insures inpatient hospital care and visits for the beneficiary. Medicare Part A covers hospital stays, room and food, medical tests, doctors' fees, skilled nursing care, hospice care, and some forms of home healthcare. Individuals are allowed to enroll on their 65th birthday and, if the individual pays into the Supplemental Security Income system for 10 years, it does not require a monthly premium. A patient may still pay some copays depending on the services required. Coverage is based on national coverage decisions as well as local decisions made by companies in each state on what is considered medically necessary.

MEDICARE PART B

Medicare Part B is part of the United States government's insurance plan that insures outpatient care, including doctors' visits, routine physicals and wellness checks, mammograms, X-rays, laboratory work, home health, physical and occupational therapy, infusion clinics, diabetes, prostate screenings, and other medically necessary and preventative services. This also includes ambulance services and durable medical equipment. Premiums must be paid, but they may be deducted from an individual's Supplemental Security Income check, as well as deductibles and copays if a service is not covered. Coverage is based on national coverage decisions as well as local decisions made by companies in each state on what is considered medically necessary.

MEDICARE PART C

Medicare Part C, also known as Medicare Advantage, is part of the United States government's insurance plan that is administered by private insurance companies that are contracted with Medicare. Medicare Part C combines elements of parts A, B, and D, and it covers health and wellness plans, vision, hearing, dental, medications, and some hospital and doctor visits. Part C typically involves a health maintenance organization, a preferred provider organization, or other similar insurance company, and a beneficiary must pay copays, premiums, and deductibles for services rendered. Typically, the patient will select a care provider from the providing company's network of physicians and professionals. An individual can enroll in Medicare Part C at age 65 or during open enrollment.

MEDICARE PART D

Medicare Part D is part of the United States government's insurance plan that assists in supporting prescription drug coverage. Medicare Part D is considered optional, but it is available to all Medicare beneficiaries who are willing to pay the fees. Coverage for Medicare Part D is provided by private companies and can be purchased by itself or can be used to supplement other plans, including Medicare Part C. Patients must pay premiums, copays, and deductibles for the plan, and they must select from pharmacies within the provider's established network. An individual can enroll in Medicare Part D at age 65 or during open enrollment.

CODING
PAYMENT POLICY
TYPES OF PAYERS THAT CODERS BILL

The purpose of medical coders is to code diagnoses and services in order to effectively bill health insurance for the costs of services. Whereas some patients pay for their medical expenses out of pocket with their own money, most patients will have one or more health plans that are billed. Most of these payers fall under three categories:

- **Commercial carriers** are private insurance companies that offer medical insurance for groups and individuals. They include organizations such as Blue Cross/Blue Shield, Aetna, and other major providers. Contracts provided by these companies cover a wide variety of services and individual plans.
- **Medicare** is the United States' primary government-funded insurance, paid for by the federal government and administered by CMS. Medicare is available to individuals older than age 65 or those who are blind, disabled, or suffering from permanent kidney failure or ESRD. Medicare is made up of multiple parts (Medicare Parts A, B, C, and D).
- **Medicaid** is an insurance assistance program sponsored at the federal and state level for low-income individuals, especially pregnant women and children. Medicaid coverage varies from state to state, but it must adhere to certain federal guidelines.

MIPS

The merit-based incentive payment system (MIPS) is one of two programs used to determine Medicare payments in order to promote improvement and innovation in clinical activities. Established in April 2015 as part of the Medicare Access and Children's Health Insurance Program Reauthorization Act, MIPS measures a participating provider's (referred to as eligible clinicians) performance based on the **quality** of performance, **promoting interoperability** by using electronic health record technology, **improvement activities** such as care coordination and patient safety, and **cost** of care. The combined aggregate score determines whether participating eligible clinicians receive an adjustment (either positive, negative, or neutral) to their Medicare reimbursement.

APMs

Alternative payment models (APMs) are one of two tracks used to determine Medicare payments for services rendered. Established in April 2015 as part of the Medicare Access and Children's Health Insurance Program Reauthorization Act, APMs are meant to ensure that patients, especially patients suffering from chronic conditions, receive care while avoiding unnecessary errors or duplication of services. Over time, providers who receive a substantial percentage of their Medicare Part B payments or see a substantial percentage of their Medicare patients through an APM can earn a 5% yearly incentive payment. Unlike MIPS, there are a wide variety of APMs available, depending on the specialty and provider type.

PLACE OF SERVICE REPORTING
PLACE OF SERVICE CODES

A place of service code is a two-digit code used on a healthcare professional's service claim document to show what setting the professional's services were provided in. The place of service code list is maintained by CMS, and it can greatly affect the reimbursement rate of the professional depending on the code used when billing Medicare, Medicaid, or private insurance. Place of service codes are divided into categories based on whether treatment takes place in a medical facility or not. Place of service codes are separate from codes used for diagnosis and procedure identification, and they are not coded alongside them.

FACILITY VS. NON-FACILITY PLACE OF SERVICE CODES

Place of service codes are divided into facility and non-facility codes. Facility codes cover services provided by hospitals, skilled nursing facilities, or ambulatory surgical centers. Non-facility codes cover all other locations.

Facility Codes	Non-facility Codes
02: Telehealth	01: Pharmacy
21: Inpatient hospital	03: School
22: On-campus outpatient hospital	04: Homeless shelter
23: Emergency room (hospital)	09: Prison/correctional facility
24: Ambulatory surgical center	11: Office
26: Military treatment facility	12: Home
31: Skilled nursing facility	13: Assisted-living facility
34: Hospice	14: Group home
41: Ambulance (land)	15: Mobile unit
42: Ambulance (air/water)	16: Temporary lodging
51: Inpatient psychiatric facility	17: Walk-in retail health clinic
52: Psychiatric facility (partial hospitalization)	20: Urgent care facility
	25: Birthing center
53: Community mental health center	32: Nursing facility
56: Residential psychiatric treatment center	33: Custodial care facility
	49: Independent clinic
61: Comprehensive inpatient rehabilitation facility	50: Federally qualified health center
	54: Intermediate care facility for individuals with intellectual disabilities
	55: Residential substance abuse treatment facility
	57: Nonresidential substance abuse treatment facility
	60: Mass immunization center
	62: Comprehensive outpatient rehabilitation facility
	65: ESRD treatment facility
	71: State/local public health clinic
	72: Rural health clinic
	81: Independent laboratory
	99: Other place of service

FRAUD AND ABUSE

FRAUD IN MEDICAL CODING

It is possible to commit fraud as a medical coder—fraud being the criminal deception of an individual or organization for financial gain. In this case, fraud involves overcharging insurance companies or falsely reporting services that were not provided. Common examples of coding fraud include the following:

- Applying a higher-paying billing code to a professional service, also known as upcoding
- Billing services provided or performed by nurses, residents, and staff under codes that are used only for a physician's duties
- Billing the components of a bundled code separately, also known as unbundling
- Billing a treatment that was performed during a single encounter as if it occurred over multiple days, also known as split billing
- Reporting a higher number of units of service than what was provided.

Ignorance of these rules will not prevent disciplinary action. Care must be taken to avoid unintentional fraud.

COMPLIANCE AUDITS

Regular audits are typically performed to ensure accurate coding, maximize quality and reimbursement of services, and to ensure compliance with proper practices and standards and preventing coding fraud. Typically, compliance audits are performed by a certified outside party. Coding audits can be either **prospective** or **retrospective.** A prospective audit is performed before a claim is fully submitted in order to catch mistakes before they're made. Retrospective audits, conversely, are performed after claims are processed, and they can typically cover a percentage of claims submitted by an individual or service provider. Failing an audit can lead to disciplinary action, either for an individual coder or for a service provider.

OIG

Established in 1976, the Office of Inspector General (OIG) is a government agency tasked with maintaining the integrity of Health and Human Services programs. Typically, this means assisting the medical industry in overseeing Medicare and Medicaid guidelines, preventing fraud and abuse, ensuring compliance, educating the public, and taking action against service providers who fail to comply with their established standards. The OIG also performs audits and provides guidelines for compliance plans that are used by medical service providers. In the event of fraud or other criminal activities, the OIG has authority to exclude individuals or organizations from receiving payment from federal healthcare programs such as Medicare and Medicaid.

OIG COMPLIANCE PLAN

An OIG compliance plan is an essential document that almost all healthcare providers and healthcare facilities use to ensure appropriate guidance and compliance with the OIG's guidelines and to minimize claim errors. Compliance plans, per the OIG's official recommendations, include seven key components, which are summarized as follows:

1. Conducting internal monitoring and auditing, including performing periodic audits for the purpose of evaluation
2. Developing and implementing clearly written compliance and practice standards
3. Designating or contracting a compliance officer or officers to monitor compliance efforts and enforce standards
4. Conducting appropriate training and education on the best practices and standards for procedures
5. Responding appropriately to violations and taking steps to correct problems
6. Developing and maintaining open lines of communication between staff and employees
7. Enforcing disciplinary standards.

NATIONAL CORRECT CODING INITIATIVE (NCCI) EDITS
NCCI

The National Correct Coding Initiative (NCCI) is a program created by the Centers for Medicare and Medicaid Services (CMS) to implement and promote correct coding methodologies and curtail improper coding at a national level. The NCCI's policies are based on current coding practices and conventions included in CPT, an analysis of standard medical practice, and local and national coverage determinations. Essentially, the NCCI helps to clarify codes that are used, decide which codes are bundled together or are kept separate, as well as show effective dates and **procedure-to-procedure (PTP)** edits of CPT procedure codes with included rationales. It is updated quarterly.

PRESENTATION OF INFORMATION

The NCCI provides coders with a method to assess whether codes should be used together or not. When using the NCCI, the information is usually presented as follows:

Heading	Column 1	Column 2	* = In Existence prior to 1996	Effective Date	Deletion Date * = No Data	Modifier 0 = Not allowed 1 = Allowed 9 = Nonapplicable	PTP Edit Rationale
Example	11042	0213T		20100701	*	0	Misuse of column 2 code with column 1 code

- **Column 1:** The payable code.
- **Column 2:** Codes not payable or usable in conjunction with the code in column 1.
- **In Existence Prior to 1996:** This column indicates if the edit existed prior to 1996, when the NCCI became standard procedure.
- **Effective Date:** The date that the edit came into effect.
- **Deletion Date:** The date that the edit was deleted (if done so).
- **Modifier:** Whether a correct coding modifier allows a code pair in columns 1 and 2 to bypass the edit. A 0 indicates it can't, a 1 indicates it can, and a 9 indicates that the edit is deleted and is no longer applicable.
- **PTP Edit Rationale**: The rationale behind the PTP edit.

NATIONAL COVERAGE DETERMINATION (NCD)

A national coverage determination (NCD) is a type of determination guideline of whether Medicare will pay for a particular item, service, or treatment. Determinations are made by CMS at the request of external parties (such as manufacturers or health plans) to determine whether the item or service is able to be used for a specific diagnosis based on **medical necessity**, e.g., if a procedure or item is considered appropriate for treatment. As the name suggests, NCDs are guidelines established at a national level, and all Medicare contractors are obligated to follow them. If the procedure is covered, then Medicare will reimburse the provider.

LOCAL COVERAGE DETERMINATION (LCD)

A local coverage determination (LCD) is a type of determination guideline of whether Medicare will pay for a particular item, service, or treatment. Unlike an NCD, an LCD has jurisdiction only within a specific region. If an NCD does not exist for a particular item or service, or an NCD requires additional definition, then it is up to a **Medicare administrative contractor (MAC)** to rule whether or not that service or item can be reimbursed based on medical necessity, thus creating an LCD within that contractor's region. Lists of LCDs are published regularly in order to provide coders with appropriate guidance.

HIPAA

Created in 1996, the Healthcare Information Portability and Accountability Act (HIPAA) is a federal law that establishes protections for sensitive health information, sets national standards for the security of electronic healthcare transactions, and institutes measures to prevent healthcare fraud and abuse. Most noticeably for medical coders, HIPAA defines privacy rules in regard to patient information and sets national standards for code sets and unique identifiers for health plans, health providers, and employers, which currently form the HCPCS, CPT, and ICD-10-CM. HIPAA's privacy rules apply to all covered entities, including doctors' offices, clinics, psychologists, dentists, nursing homes, pharmacies, health insurance companies, and healthcare clearinghouses.

PRIVACY GUIDELINES

HIPAA stipulates that only the **minimum necessary** amount of a patient's particular medical and personal information should be shared or provided to satisfy a specific medical purpose and only to those who require it. For example, a nurse working with an HIV-positive patient should not share that patient's HIV status with a peer while the nurse is off duty.

This standard does have some exceptions; information may be disclosed if:

- It is required to provide treatment.
- It is disclosed to the subject of the information.
- It is pursuant to an authorization of an individual.
- It is required for compliance with HIPAA's rules.
- It is disclosed to the Department of Health and Human Services for purposes of enforcement.
- It is required by other laws.

ADVANCE BENEFICIARY NOTICES (ABNs)

An advance beneficiary notice (ABN) is a standardized, one-page Medicare form used to notify a patient that a procedure, treatment, or service may not be covered by Medicare. An ABN explains why Medicare may deny the procedure or procedures, and it is used to protect the provider's financial interests by creating a paper trail if Medicare denies reimbursement. An ABN alone is not sufficient; the patient should also be provided with a specific explanation as to why a service may be denied. An ABN also cannot be used to bill a patient for additional fees beyond what Medicare reimburses. ABNs may not be used for emergency or urgent care situations.

RELATIVE VALUE UNITS (RVUs)

Relative value units (RVUs) are a measure of value established for Medicare as part of the **resource-based relative value scale (RBRVS)**. The intention was to create a stable and non-variable rate for Medicare payments for physician services, rather than the more inconsistent system that existed before. RVUs themselves have no financial value; instead, they inform how much a particular service is worth (for example, a service with an RVU of 3 is worth three times as much as a service with an RVU of 1). RVUs cover three different factors: the **physician's work**, which represents the time, skill, and difficulty of the service provided; the **practice expense**, which reflects the costs of personnel, supplies, and overhead; and the **liability/malpractice expense** for the purposes of insurance.

CALCULATION

The RBRVS is a formula that is used to calculate how much Medicare reimburses a provider for procedures. CMS annually publishes this information on its website and provides comprehensive listings for all RVUs. The formula used for calculating reimbursement is as follows:

$$[(W\ RVU \times W\ GPCI) + (PE\ RVU \times PE\ GPCI) + (MP\ RVU \times MP\ GPCI)] \times \text{conversion factor.}$$

- **RVU**: the relative value unit for work performed (W), physician's expense ([PE] facility or non-facility), and malpractice liability (MP)
- **GPCI**: the **geographic practice cost index**, which varies based on the location of the practice
- **Conversion factor:** a fixed dollar amount used to translate the resulting formula into fees.

CPC Practice Test

1. A patient undergoes surgery with anesthesia and is arousable with painful stimulation. What is the level of sedation the patient MOST likely received?

    a. Moderate sedation
    b. Minimal sedation
    c. General anesthesia
    d. Deep sedation

2. A patient presents to physical therapy status post repair of a complete rotator cuff tear in the right shoulder due to a fall. After applying ice to the shoulder for 8 minutes, the physical therapist performs a soft-tissue massage to the infraspinatus muscle that lasts 23 minutes. Just prior to discharge, the therapist spends 20 minutes instructing the patient on isokinetic exercises to help improve range of motion. Which CPT and ICD-10-CM code(s) should be used to accurately describe encounter?

    a. 97010, 97140, 97530, S46.011A, W19.XXXA
    b. 97110, 97140, 97010, Z48.89, S46.091A, W19.XXXA
    c. 97010, 97140 x 2, 97530, M75.121
    d. 97110, 97140 x 2, 97010, S46.011D, W19.XXXD

3. A diaphragm resection and repair are done using a biologic mesh to reduce the formation of adhesions. Which procedure code should be reported?

    a. 39501
    b. 39560
    c. 39561
    d. 39599

4. An established 27-year-old female patient is seen with complaints of fatigue and muscle aches that began 3 days ago. The physician draws two vials of blood, collects a urine sample, and performs a pregnancy test. The patient is instructed to drink 8 ounces of water daily, rest, and follow up in 3 days for her results. What CPT codes should be reported for this encounter?

    a. 99213, 81025, 36410, 81005
    b. 99212, 81025, 36416, 81007
    c. 99213, 81025, 36415, 81002
    d. 99212, 81025, 36410x2, 99000, 81020

5. If past family and social history is not documented for the evaluation and management of a new patient, what is the highest level of service that can be coded?

    a. 99202
    b. 99213
    c. 99201
    d. 99212

6. Code the following adverse effect:

Initial encounter of drug-induced tremors that was caused by Cyclosporin the patient takes for anemia. The anemia is caused by a current diagnosis of colon cancer.

a. D63.0, C18.9, T45.1X5A, G25.1
b. G25.1, T45.1X5A, C18.9, D63.0
c. T45.1X5A, G25.1, C18.9, D63.0
d. C18.9, D63.0, G25.1, T45.1X5A

7. Under the oversight of the pediatrician, a nurse reviews the vaccine and allergy history of a 13-year-old established patient just prior to administering a live varicella virus vaccine subcutaneously. What procedure code(s) should be reported?

a. 99211-25, 90716, 90471
b. 90716, 90471
c. 90716, 90460
d. 99211-25, 90716, 90460

8. A complete pulmonary function test using a body plethysmograph is performed on a patient in conjunction with spirometry. After reviewing the results, a provider suspects the presence of an obstructive disease and administers a bronchodilating medicine just prior to repeating the test to reevaluate the expiratory flow rate. Which code(s) should be reported?

a. 99212-25, 94726, 94060-76
b. 99212-25, 94726, 94010-51, 94060-51
c. 94726, 94060-51
d. 94726, 94060

9. An established patient presents complaining of clumpy, white discharge for 3 days. A vaginal exam reveals an old tampon, which is removed. Diflucan is sent to the pharmacy, instructions given, and the patient is told to follow up in 1 week. How would the provider code the visit?

a. 57415, T19.2XXA, N89.8
b. 57415, 99212-25, T19.2XXA
c. 99213, T19.2XXA, N89.8
d. 99213, N89.8, T19.2XXA

10. Which service is NOT included in the central nervous system assessment?

a. Review of an advance care plan
b. Clinical dementia rating
c. Prescription for an opioid
d. Discussion of suicidal intentions

11. Code the following surgical note:

> Patient is seen for an epidural injection into the following three levels: L3-L4, L4-L5 and L5-S1.
>
> A 22-gauge spinal needle is inserted into the zygapophyseal joint using fluoroscopic guidance. After confirming the needles placement at L3-L4 on the left side, 0.5 cc of a local anesthetic is injected into the joint. The whole process is repeated on the left side at the other two levels. The procedure was completed without any complications.

a. 64493-LT, 64494-LT, 64495-LT
b. 0216T-LT, 0217T-LT, 0218T-LT
c. 64493-LT, 64494-59-LT, 64495-59-LT
d. 62323

12. Code the following physician's note:

> A 14-year-old established patient is seen with mother to evaluate five 2 cm superficial lacerations to the left wrist. Patient admits to suicidal thoughts. Lacerations were treated with Steri-Strips. Patient and mother counseled on suicide prevention and told to follow up with psych.

a. 12004, S61.512A, R45.851
b. 12004, S61.512A, T14.91XA
c. 99214, S61.512A, T14.91XA
d. 99213, S61.512A, R45.851

13. A physician performs an esophagogastroduodenoscopy on a patient who has GERD. A single tissue sample is obtained from the upper gastrointestinal tract using biopsy forceps. A reflux test was also done and a bravo capsule temporarily attached to the esophageal wall to monitor pH levels. What procedures should the physician report?

a. 43239, 91034
b. 43235, 91035
c. 43235, 91034
d. 43239, 91035

14. Assign the CPT codes for the following surgical note:

> A patient who is confirmed to have lymphoma is placed under general anesthesia. A flexible bronchoscope is first inserted through the oral cavity to determine if the primary carcinoma has spread to the lung tissue. No lesions are observed in the bronchus, and the bronchoscope is removed. An incision is then made in the parasternal second left intercostal space, thus exposing the anterior mediastinal lymph nodes. Tissue samples from the lymph nodes are removed without complication. The incision is closed with sutures, and the patient is discharged to recovery.

a. 39010, 31623-51
b. 39010, 31622-51
c. 39402, 31622-51
d. 39402, 31623-51

15. A patient who is experiencing rectal bleeding has a colonoscopy. Prior to the procedure, the provider administers general anesthesia. What CPT code(s) should be reported?

    a. 45382, 00811
    b. 45378-47
    c. 45378, 00811-47
    d. 45382

16. To rule out malignancy, a provider collects two biopsies from the right thyroid nodule using a large bore needle that is inserted through the skin. Which CPT code(s) should be reported?

    a. 10021, 10041
    b. 60100
    c. 10021, 10041-59
    d. 60100, 60100-59

17. A 79-year-old female patient is admitted to a skilled nursing facility for continued monitoring as she completes her course of antibiotics for bronchitis. Upon admission, a nurse practitioner spends 20 minutes with the patient, performing an evaluation of recovery and rebuilding of stamina. On day 3, the patient's physician completes an initial comprehensive assessment and determines the patient is recovering well on her current dosage of antibiotics. What CPT code should be reported on day 3?

    a. 99304
    b. 99305
    c. 99309
    d. 99310

18. Which term describes a procedure in which real-time moving images of an organ are displayed on a screen so that a physician can examine its function and/or structure?

    a. Magnetic resonance imaging
    b. Tomography
    c. Fluoroscopy
    d. Computed tomography

19. During surgery to remove a malignant melanoma from the intestinal tract, one frozen section is sent for pathological consultation to confirm an adequate excision of the margins. A second specimen is also sent, which requires frozen sections on two tissue blocks. What CPT code(s) should the pathologist report?

    a. 88331, 88331, 88332
    b. 88331, 88332, 88332
    c. 88329, 88331, 88332, 88332
    d. 88331, 88332

20. Which patient is receiving critical care services?

    a. A 47-year-old female with a history of unrepaired chronic heart disease and anemia has an oxygen saturation level of 80. She is put on a nasal cannula and given a blood transfusion to improve her oxygen-carrying capacity and oxygen saturation level.

    b. A 60-year-old male is admitted with an acute chronic heart failure exacerbation causing hypoxic respiratory failure. The patient is intubated, sedated, and started on 50 mg of ertapenem for a potential lung infection.

    c. A 67-year-old female receives chronic ventilator therapy after a cerebral infarction that caused hemorrhage in the brain.

    d. A 93-year-old male is admitted to the intensive care unit for monitoring after a coronary angioplasty procedure that was performed to relieve symptoms of atherosclerosis.

21. If a cardiologist bills an electrocardiogram (93010) in the emergency department and then follows up with the patient a week later for arteriosclerosis, he should bill an established patient E/M.

    a. True

    b. False

22. A low-risk obstetrical patient is told to come in for weekly ultrasounds in her first trimester. This is an example of what?

    a. Fraud

    b. Abuse

    c. Waste

    d. Misuse

23. CPT code 99135 is an example of a qualifying circumstance.

    a. True

    b. False

24. A laboratory receives a pap smear as a screening for a patient's annual gynecological exam. A thin-layer preparation screened by an automated system with manual rescreening is performed. A pathologist interprets the results and confirms a diagnosis of high-grade squamous intraepithelial lesion. What should the laboratory report?

    a. G0148, G0141, Z12.4 R87.613

    b. G0148, R87.610

    c. 88175, Z12.4

    d. 88175, 88141, Z01.419, R87.613

25. A surgeon performs a craniectomy to excise a meningioma located above the tentorium cerebelli. During the procedure, an extradural hematoma is noted and removed via the same craniectomy site. How should the surgeon report the procedure?

    a. 61312-22

    b. 61512, 61312-59

    c. 61519, 61314-51

    d. 61512

26. A patient is admitted for chemical burns caused by a leaky car battery. The physician diagnoses the patient with second- and third-degree burns on the right hand and second-degree burns on the left hand. The physician follows up with the patient 3 days later and performs a detailed examination. His findings include an infection that has developed on the right hand as a result of the burn. The patient is started on antibiotics. Code this encounter.

    a. 99232, L08.9, T23.201S, T23.361S, T23.301S, T23.202A, T54.2X4A
    b. 99231, T23.201A, T23.361A, T23.301A, T23.202A, T54.2X4A, L08.9
    c. 99232, T23.701A, T23.662A, T54.21XA, L08.9
    d. 99231, L08.9, T23.T23.701S, T23.662A, T54.21XS

27. When it comes to documentation, what is NOT included in the history of present illness?

    a. Quantity
    b. Duration
    c. Timing
    d. Quality

28. A 15-year-old male patient is seen in the emergency department due to a dislocated left elbow, caused by a fall from his skateboard. The physician performs a comprehensive physical evaluation to check for other injuries before manually realigning the dislocation and placing a splint from the shoulder to wrist. The patient is informed to follow up in 4 weeks. Which CPT and ICD-10-CM codes should the emergency department report?

    a. 24600-LT, S53.105A, V00.131A
    b. 99283, 24600-LT, S53.105A, V00.131A
    c. 24600-LT, 29105, S53.195A, V00.131A
    d. 99282-57, 24600-LT, S53.105A, V00.131A

29. A surgeon performs a posterior fusion on the L2-L5 of the spine due to degenerative disc disease. What CPT and ICD-10-CM code(s) should be reported?

    a. 22612, 22614 x 2, M51.36
    b. 22800, M51.37
    c. 22553, M51.37
    d. 22612, 22614 x 3, M51.36

30. A provider places a catheter on the right side of the heart chamber via an incision made on the lower left side of the patient's chest while performing a transcatheter mitral valve replacement. How should this encounter be coded?

    a. 33430
    b. 0483T, 93451
    c. 0484T, 93451-59
    d. 0484T

31. A 92-year old female with Medicare part A coverage receives ongoing hospice care due to dementia. She goes to a physician's office to receive closed treatment of a hip dislocation following a fall. No anesthesia was used. How should the provider submit this claim?

    a. 27250, S73.003A, W19.XXXA
    b. 27250-GW, S73.003A, W19.XXXA
    c. 27250-GW, 99202-25, S73.003A, W19.XXXA
    d. 27250, 99213-25, S73.003A, W19.XXXA

32. If a provider documents in an assessment that a patient is obese, but the BMI extracted from the chart is consistent with morbid obesity, what should be reported on the claim?

    a. Morbid obesity
    b. Morbid obesity and the appropriate BMI
    c. Obesity
    d. Obesity and the appropriate BMI

33. Code the excision of a large goiter extending into the chest cavity using a transthoracic approach.

    a. 32900
    b. 32140
    c. 21602
    d. 60270

34. Which is NOT a type of injection through which contrast is administered?

    a. Intramuscular
    b. Intravascular
    c. Intra-articular
    d. Intrathecal

35. Modifier 50 is not an appropriate modifier to append on CPT code 52000.

    a. True
    b. False

36. A patient is scheduled for a total knee replacement. The assigned anesthesiologist performs a femoral nerve block using an ultrasound machine just prior to entering the operating room to aid in postoperative pain control. Once in the operating room, general anesthesia is administered to the patient. What CPT code(s) should the anesthesiologist report?

    a. 01402
    b. 01400, 01991, 76942
    c. 01402, 64447-59, 76942
    d. 01400, 01991-59

37. Which of the four chambers in the heart receives deoxygenated blood from the body through the vena cava?

    a. Right atrium
    b. Left ventricle
    c. Right ventricle
    d. Left atrium

38. Code the following procedure note:

A selective catheter is placed into the thoracic aorta, where it is then manipulated into the left coronary artery and followed through into the right common carotid artery. Contrast injections are made, and digital imaging is performed. Upon completion, the catheter is removed, pressure is applied at the puncture site, and the patient is discharged.

a. 36217
b. 36215, 36216-59
c. 36216
d. 36200, 36215, 36216-59

39. What would NOT be included in critical care services?

a. CPR
b. Pulse oximetry
c. Gastric intubation
d. Ventilator management

40. If the dermatologist removes 17 skin tags from a patient's lumbar using local anesthesia and a sharp blade, which CPT code(s) should be reported?

a. 11200, 11201-51, 00300
b. 11200, 11201
c. 11200
d. 11200, 11201, 00300

41. A patient presents to urgent care with complaints of a sore throat, a temperature of 100.2, and pain while urinating. The provider examines the patient and collects a throat swab and urine sample. The following codes are then entered on the patients claim: R30.9, R07.0, R50.9, N39.0, J03.8, and B95.3. What code(s) should be removed?

a. B95.3
b. N39.0, J03.8, B95.3
c. R30.9, R07.0 and R50.9
d. R30.9, R07.0

42. A physician inserts a chest tube through the right chest wall and into the pleural cavity to release trapped air in a 19-year-old patient with recurring pneumothorax. A second physician assists in providing moderate sedation. In total, the procedure took 8 minutes. What ICD-10-CM and CPT codes should the provider report?

a. 32551, 99156-59, J93.9
b. 32550, J93.9
c. 32551, J93.83
d. 32550-62, 99156, J93.83

43. A provider documents that he spent 20 minutes with a patient. Based on this, an E/M can be chosen solely based on time.

a. True
b. False

44. What is NOT a function of the kidneys?

a. Propel urine
b. Filter blood
c. Remove waste
d. Regulate blood pressure

45. A 59-year-old male patient presents for a routine colonoscopy. During the procedure, a polyp is discovered. What is the proper ICD-10-CM coding for this encounter?

a. Z12.11, K63.5
b. Z12.11
c. K63.5, Z12.11
d. K63.5

46. A 34-year-old established male patient presents for treatment to his lower back. He reports exacerbated symptoms due to lifting heavy materials at work. The osteopath performs a problem-focused history and exam followed by manipulative treatment to the lumbar and sacral region of the spine. What procedure(s) should the osteopath report?

a. 98940
b. 98925
c. 99212-25, 97140x2
d. 99212-25, 98925

47. A 55-year-old patient is admitted into the hospital for dialysis to treat ESRD. On day 13, the admitting physician spends 25 minutes discussing new management options for the patient's hypertension before sending a nurse to initiate the hemodialysis procedure. What CPT and ICD-10-CM codes should be reported?

a. 90935, N18.6, Z99.2
b. 90937, 99232, I10, N18.6, Z99.2
c. 90937, I12.0, N18.6, Z99.2
d. 99232, I12.0, N18.6, Z99.2

48. A physician performs a simple repair on a Medicare patient who comes in with a 2.7 cm cut, an open wound, on the neck. The repair is made with Dermabond. Which CPT code(s) should be reported?

a. G0168
b. 12002
c. 12002, G0168
d. 99213-25, G0168

49. A sternal closure using sutures is considered inclusive to CPT 33255 and should not be reported separately.

a. True
b. False

50. A 22-year-old patient presents with a 5.5 cm gaping laceration on the right forearm and a 2 cm superficial laceration on the right wrist caused by a table saw. A local anesthetic is injected around both laceration sites. The physician irrigates the laceration on the wrist before closing the wound with a tissue adhesive and then performs an extensive cleaning and single-layer closure with sutures on the forearm. What should be coded for this encounter?

 a. 12032, 97597, G0168, S41.111A, S61.411A, W31.2XXA
 b. 12001, 12032-59, S61.411A, S41.111A, W31.2XXA
 c. 12032, 12001-59, S41.111A, S61.411A, W31.2XXA
 d. 12032, S41.111A, S61.411A, W31.2XXA

51. A patient is referred to a radiology clinic with a diagnosis of chest bruising. A radiologist who works for the clinic performs a 3-view x-ray on the patient's ribcage bilaterally. The radiologist interprets images and determines that there is a right-sided stress fracture to one rib. Which ICD-10-CM and CPT codes should be reported for this encounter?

 a. 71110-26, M84.48XA
 b. 71110-26, S22.31XA
 c. 71110, S22.31XA
 d. 71110, M84.48XA

52. A patient is having difficulties breast-feeding and receives a lactation consultation by a certified lactation consultant under the general supervision of a mid-level practitioner. How should this service be reported?

 a. 98966
 b. 99211
 c. 99078
 d. 98960

53. Code the following procedure note:

> A 45-year-old female was referred for a urodynamics study due to complaints of bladder pain and weak urination. The provider places a rectal catheter simultaneously with a urethral catheter and begins to fill the bladder with water. Using calibrated equipment, cytometry was done with a medium fill rate of 40 cc/minute. A strong desire to void occurred at 84 cc, and the patient is instructed to void. The provider determines that the maximum urinary flow rate is 12 cc per second with a voiding time of 45 seconds and a voided volume of 102 cc. She voided with a sustained detrusor pressure. An abdominal pressure measurement was also taken, indicating no urinary leaking with abdominal straining. EMG patches were placed on the anal sphincter and found to be elevated with increased intra-abdominal pressure. All catheters and EMG patches were removed, and the procedure was completed without complications. A report will be forwarded to the referring provider, who will provide the interpretation of the results to the patient.

 a. 51726-TC, 51784-59-TC, 51797-59-TC, 51741-59-TC
 b. 51726-TC, 51784-51-TC, 51797-51-TC
 c. 51728-TC, 51784-TC, 51797-TC
 d. 51728-TC, 51784-TC, 51797-TC, 51741-TC

54. CPT code 11102 is a column 2 code that has an NCCI edit of 1 when paired with CPT code 11402. How would this be interpreted?

    a. The two codes are inclusive of each other and can never be billed together.
    b. If being billed together, only report one unit of each.
    c. The two codes are exclusive of each other and can never be billed together.
    d. The two codes can be billed together with an appropriate modifier.

55. Which is NOT part of the upper respiratory tract?

    a. Pharynx
    b. Nasal cavity
    c. Larynx
    d. Trachea

56. The laboratory collected blood to test the patient's carbon dioxide, chloride, potassium, sodium, and glucose levels. Select the CPT codes that the laboratory will report.

    a. 80052-52
    b. 80051, 82947
    c. 80051, 80053
    d. 80051, 82947-59

57. An established 4-year-old patient is seen by her pediatrician with complaints of pain in her left wrist after falling. The pediatrician determines the wrist is sprained and applies a splint that will keep the wrist from being able to move. The patient's mother is told to follow up if symptoms worsen. What code(s) should be reported for this encounter?

    a. 99212-25, 29126, E1805
    b. 29125, S8451
    c. 99212-25, 29125, S8451
    d. 29126, E1805

58. The appendix is removed through an abdominal incision due to metastatic colon malignancy. How should this be reported?

    a. 44970, C78.5
    b. 44970, C18.9, C78.5
    c. 44950, C78.5
    d. 44950, C78.5, C18.9

59. What is the main role of the tonsils?

    a. Remove bacteria that enter the body through the nose and/or mouth
    b. Trigger the formation of antibodies
    c. Filter lymph and form lymphocytes
    d. Secrete antibodies to destroy ingested microbes

60. The base unit for anesthesia CPT code 00600 is 10 units. If an anesthesiologist spends 105 minutes in the procedure room with a patient, how many units should be reported for reimbursement?

    a. 11 units
    b. 12 units
    c. 14 units
    d. 17 units

61. A physician documents a comprehensive electrophysiologic evaluation with an unsuccessful attempted induction of arrhythmia. Upon review, the bundle-of-His recording is missing. What code(s) should be reported?

a. 96320
b. 93610, 93602, 93612, 93603, 93618
c. 93620-52
d. 93619-52

62. It is appropriate to use a HCPCS Level II G code, as opposed to a CPT code, to report a screening service performed on an asymptomatic patient.

a. True
b. False

63. Which term describes a migraine that is unmanageable with treatment?

a. A migraine with aura
b. Status migrainosus
c. Intractable migraine
d. Classical migraine

64. Which option would best fall under a level II HCPC code?

a. Radiation treatment management
b. Diagnostic colonoscopy
c. A malignant neoplasm
d. Advanced life support

65. A young man is triaged in the emergency room after sustaining multiple injuries in a car accident. The physician performs the following limited exams with image documentation: an abdominal and retroperitoneal ultrasound, a transthoracic echocardiography, and a chest ultrasound. He indicates in his report that all findings are normal. What charges should the provider submit to the insurance company?

a. 93304-TC, 76700-TC, 76770-TC, 76604-TC
b. 93308-26, 76705-26, 76775-26, 76604-26
c. 99308, 76705-59, 76770-59, 76604-59
d. 93304-26, 76705-26, 76775-26, 76604-26

66. A 45-year-old female patient with urinary incontinence is treated by means of a Burch procedure. The patient is morbidly obese. What CPT and ICD-10-CM codes should be reported by the surgeon?

a. 51840, R32
b. 51841, R32, E66.8
c. 51840, R32, E66.8
d. 51841, R32

67. Which procedure uses a thin tube to examine the abdominal organs through a small incision in the belly?

a. Gastroscopy
b. Laparoscopy
c. Endoscopy
d. Laparotomy

68. Assign the appropriate CPT codes for the following surgical note:

A 15-year-old patient is being treated for obstructive sleep apnea and adenoid tissue hypertrophy. After being placed under general anesthesia, a dental mirror is placed in the oropharynx to allow visualization of the nasopharynx. Suction electrocautery is used to remove the adenoid tissue that regrew after the initial adenoidectomy. Attention is then turned to the tonsils. The plane of tissue between the tonsillar capsule and the underlying muscles are cauterized, and the tonsils are removed. Bleeding is controlled by silver nitrate and gauze packing. Procedure is completed without complications, and patient is discharged to recovery.

a. 42826, 42831-59, J35.2, G47.33
b. 42999, G47.33, J35.2
c. 42826, 42836-51, J35.2, G47.33
d. 42821, G47.33, J35.2

69. Which type of anesthesia is NOT separately reportable?

a. Metacarpal blocks
b. Monitored anesthesia care
c. Spinal anesthesia
d. Regional anesthesia

70. What is NOT a condition related to the thyroid gland?

a. Toxic adenoma
b. Graves' disease
c. Hashimoto's disease
d. Acosta disease

71. Assign the appropriate procedure and diagnosis codes for a biopsy of a posterior mediastinal mass that was obtained through an incision at the base of the neck.

a. 39000, D38.3
b. 39401, D49.89
c. 39000, R22.2
d. 39401, R22.1

72. A 74-year-old patient is admitted into observational care after a comprehensive history and exam confirms pneumonia. She has a medical history of being HIV positive. How should this be reported?

a. 99235, B20, J18.9
b. 99236, B20, J18.9
c. 99235, J18.9, B20
d. 99236, J18.9, B20

73. **A female patient presents to her obstetrical office 32-weeks pregnant for a bi-weekly ultrasound. Code the following technician's report:**

> Fetal views obtained via transabdominal ultrasound as follows:
> BPD: 82 mm
> Femur Length: 63 mm
> Head Circumference: 288 mm
> Abdominal Circumference: 270 mm
> BPP 8/8
> NST from 11:15 to 12:17, showing 160 BPM and positive movement activity
> Doppler shows adequate systolic and diastolic flow velocities of the fetal umbilical artery.

   a. 76816, 76818, 76820
   b. 76815-TC, 76819-TC, 76820-TC
   c. 76815, 78819, 76820
   d. 76816-TC, 76816-TC, 76820-TC

74. **An obstetrical patient carrying twins is seen. The physician performs a fetal nonstress test on each fetus. How should the CPT code(s) be reported?**

   a. 59025, 59025-59
   b. 59025
   c. 59025-76
   d. 59025-22

75. **Which antibody test results indicate a current, acute infection?**

   a. IgG positive, IgM positive
   b. IgG positive, IgM positive
   c. IgG negative, IgM negative
   d. IgM positive, IgG negative

76. **A patient is seen with complaints of recurring infections in the foreskin. The physician recommends circumcision to help improve penile hygiene. The patient agrees, a local anesthetic is injected into the penis, and the procedure is completed by clamping the foreskin and trimming the excess skin. How should the physician report the encounter?**

   a. 54150, 64450, Z41.2, Z87.2
   b. 54150-52, 64450, N48.89
   c. 54150, N48.29
   d. 54150-52, Z41.2, Z87.2

77. **A female patient experiencing swollen lymph nodes is seen for a follow-up to discuss the results of her open axillary biopsy that occurred last week. The results are positive for diffuse large cell lymphoma. The patient is given multiple treatment options, including success rates, risks, and side effects. She opts to begin radiation treatment next week. What CPT and ICD-10-CM codes should the provider report for this visit?**

   a. 99213-24, C83.84
   b. 99214, C85.94
   c. 99212-24, 25, 99024, C83.34
   d. 99024, C85.84

78. An 8-year year old female is seen by her pediatrician for an allergic reaction to a bee sting. The pediatrician administers 0.3 mg of epinephrine intramuscularly. Which code(s) should be reported?

    a. 96372, J0171 (3 units)
    b. J0171 (3 units)
    c. 99212, J0171
    d. 99213-25, 96372, J0171 (3 units)

79. What would be considered a sequela to an injury?

    a. Foreign body removal from a laceration
    b. Removal of an external fixation device
    c. Prescription drug management
    d. Chronic pain persisting after an injury has healed

80. A 74-year-old male patient recently had a bone marrow transplant due to aplastic anemia. At his follow-up visit with the doctor, his blood is drawn and sent to the laboratory to determine if the engraftment was successful. The laboratory evaluates the immature reticulocyte fraction (IRF) using an automated cell counter and total reticulocyte by way of a manual count. What codes should the laboratory report?

    a. 85046, D61.9, Z79.81
    b. 85046, D61.9
    c. 85046, 85044, D61.9
    d. 85046, 85044, D61.9, Z94.81

81. Anesthesiologist A begins providing services at 7:02 but is relieved at 8:47 by Anesthesiologist Z. If the recorded end time for anesthesia services is 11:32, which statement is be true?

    a. Anesthesiologist Z would report 4.5 hours of anesthesia time.
    b. Anesthesiologist A would report 1.75 hours, and Anesthesiologist Z would report 2.75 hours of anesthesia time.
    c. Anesthesiologist A would report 4.5 hours of anesthesia time.
    d. Both anesthesiologists would separately report 4.5 hours of anesthesia time.

82. The relative value units of a procedure are based on how much effort is involved, expenses that the practice will incur, and the level of risk associated with it.

    a. True
    b. False

83. An extracapsular cataract extraction procedure was performed on a patient with a clouded and discolored lens. The physician uses iris hooks in the right pupil to ensure safe and controlled access to the cataract and blue staining dye to visualize the capsulorhexis. Using suction, the existing lens capsule is removed, and an intraocular lens is inserted. What should the physician report?

    a. 66982-RT, H27.8
    b. 66984-RT, H18.891
    c. 66982-RT, Q12.8
    d. 66984-RT, H26.8

84. Dr. Black orders a hepatitis panel for a patient who has recently returned from traveling abroad and is now experiencing lower abdominal pain. The laboratory completed a hepatitis A antibody test, hepatitis B core antibody test, and a hepatitis C antibody test. Select the CPT and the ICD-10-CM codes that the laboratory will report.

    a. 80074, R10.30
    b. 80074-52, R10.30
    c. 86709, 86705, 86803, R10.31, R10.32
    d. 86709, 86705, 86803, R10.30

85. Which is NOT a violation of Health Insurance Portability and Accountability Act (HIPAA)?

    a. An encrypted laptop is stolen from a physician's vehicle.
    b. An employee drops off patient records on a physician's porch.
    c. A hospital with a multilayered cybersecurity defense experiences a data breach by a cybercriminal.
    d. An office does not perform a risk assessment of electronic health information.

86. An established female patient presents to a video conference with her internist with complaints of a nonproductive cough. She receives 15 minutes of counseling about the symptoms of COVID-19 and is directed to an unaffiliated testing site. What CPT and ICD-10-CM codes should be reported?

    a. 99442, R05, Z20.828
    b. 99442, R05
    c. 99213-95, R05
    d. 99213-95, R05, Z20.828

87. Based on the following documentation, what would the overall medical decision-making (MDM) be?

    Number of diagnosis or management options: Minimal
    Amount and complexity of data: Moderate
    Level of Risk: Moderate

    a. Straightforward
    b. Low complexity
    c. Moderate complexity
    d. High complexity

88. A patient with a stab wound to the chest was taken to the operating room and put under general anesthesia for a thoracotomy. The anesthesiologist should report CPT 00520 with the total number of time units spent providing face-to-face care with the patient.

    a. True
    b. False

89. A patient develops an infection within the global period of a knee replacement. It is determined that the infection originated from the incision site and needs to be surgically removed. Which modifier should be appended to the secondary surgery?

    a. 58
    b. 78
    c. 79
    d. 25

90. Which service would NOT be covered under Medicare part A?

    a. Observation hospital care
    b. Inpatient hospital care
    c. Home health care
    d. Hospice care

91. What would NOT be included in a global obstetrical package?

    a. A patient with anemia comes in to check hemoglobin levels.
    b. A patient complains of flu-like symptoms and is prescribed an antibiotic.
    c. Contraception following delivery is discussed at length.
    d. Sutures are removed from a first-degree perineal laceration during the delivery.

92. A patient tests positive for coronavirus (SARS-CoV-2) and bronchitis after presenting with a cough. What diagnosis code(s) should be reported?

    a. J40, B97.29, R05
    b. U07.1, J40
    c. U07.1, J40, Z20.828
    d. J40, B97.29, Z20.828

93. If all the following statements were documented by the anesthesiologist in one record, which would be chosen as the start time for anesthesia services?

    a. Medical history and vital signs for the patient are obtained prior to the surgery.
    b. Propofol is administered to the patient intravenously.
    c. A pulse oximeter is attached to the patient's finger while in the operating room.
    d. Request for services is received for an operation that begins in 1 hour.

94. A patient with right knee pain is seen in a physician's office for an x-ray. Anteroposterior and lateral views of the right knee were obtained by the technician, and images confirm right knee pain secondary to degenerative osteoarthritis. Which CPT and ICD-10-CM code(s) should be reported?

    a. 73561-TC-RT, M17.11, M25.561
    b. 73560-26-RT, M17.11, M25.561
    c. 73560-RT, M17.11
    d. 73560-TC-RT, M17.11

95. The CPT code 76805 requires that multiple elements of the exam be documented, such as the evaluation of the amniotic fluid, umbilical cord insertion site, and placental location. If the provider documents most elements, he/she can bill the CPT code 76805.

    a. True
    b. False

96. A 39-year-old female patient has developed a diaphragmatic hernia after an episode of domestic violence. The surgeon repairs the hernia through an incision into the abdomen. The patient is later discharged with no complications. How should this encounter be reported?

    a. 39541, K44.0, T74.11XA, Y07.9
    b. 39540, K44.9, T76.11XA
    c. 39541, K44.0, T76.11XA
    d. 39540, K44.9, T74.11XA, Y07.9

97. A mammogram is done on a patient who has a lump on her right breast at 4 o'clock and a lump in her left breast at 6 o'clock. What CPT and ICD-10-CM code(s) should be reported?

    a. 77067, D49.3
    b. 77065-50, N63.13, N63.20
    c. 77067, D48.61, D48.62
    d. 77066, N63.14, N63.25

98. V codes are related to which procedures/products?

    a. Durable medical equipment
    b. Orthotic procedures
    c. Enteral therapy
    d. Hearing services

99. Which statement is true regarding the diaphragm?

    a. It is a collection of organs held together by connective tissue.
    b. It forms tendons, ligaments, cartilage, and fat.
    c. It performs an important function in blood flow.
    d. It separates the thoracic cavity from the abdominal cavity.

100. Which condition would describe a patient with a physical status modifier of P3?

    a. Multiple organ dysfunction
    b. Poorly controlled diabetes
    c. A recent myocardial infarction
    d. Sepsis

101. A new, 29-year-old female patient is seen for a preventative visit and receives counseling that totals 30 minutes about contraceptive management. How would the provider code the CPT code(s) for this visit?

    a. 99385, 99402-25
    b. 99385, 99203-25
    c. 99385, 99355
    d. 99385

102. Diagnostic endoscopy is always inclusive to a surgical endoscopy.

    a. True
    b. False

103. A patient with a history of colon cancer was treated with radiation therapy. CT scans and blood tests show the malignancy has been eradicated. The patient is directed to take 81 mg of aspirin daily over the course of the next year to help prevent reoccurrence of the malignancy. What ICD-10-CM code(s) should be reported by the provider on subsequent visits related to this patient's condition?

    a. Z48.3, C18.9
    b. C18.9
    c. Z08, Z85.038
    d. Z85.038

104. A primary care physician is requesting a second opinion to determine which strain of Ebolavirus the patient has. The specimen is sent to a pathologist, who carefully examines it. A written report is sent promptly back to the primary care physician, confirming Zaire Ebolavirus and recommending immediate isolation and emergency care. What code should be reported by the pathologist?

    a. 80502
    b. 99241
    c. 80500
    d. 99201

105. If a patient is receiving hospice care in a physician's office, which place of service code should be reported on the claim?

    a. 34
    b. 11
    c. 71
    d. 62

106. A male patient with cancerous cells in his right bronchus is given 150 mg of porfimer sodium via a single and slow intravenous injection and told to return to the office in 3 days. Upon his return, the physician enters the right bronchus by means of a bronchoscope and activates LED for a total of 38 minutes to destroy the cancer cells. What should the physician report?

    a. 96573, 96409, J9600x2
    b. 31641, 96570, 96571, J9600x2
    c. 96573, J9600x2
    d. 31641, 96570, 96571, 96409, J9600x2

107. A 72-year-old patient is admitted due to atrial fibrillation. A comprehensive electrophysiology study is completed with fluoroscopic guidance, followed by a cardiac catheter ablation during the same procedure. The procedure took 22 minutes, and the patient was moderately sedated. Which CPT codes should the cardiologist report?

    a. 93650, 93619-26-59, 77001, 99152, 99153
    b. 93650, 93619-26-59, 99152
    c. 93656, 99152
    d. 93656, 77001, 99152, 99153

108. A female patient with type II diabetes, asthma, and hypertension is admitted with complaints of chest pain. Testing rules out heart attack and other underlying conditions as the cause. Which diagnosis codes should be listed on the discharge note?

    a. R07.9, E11.9, J45.909, I10
    b. Z03.89
    c. E11.69, J45.909, I10, R07.9
    d. E11.69, J45.909, I10, Z03.89

109. A physician performs a thyroidectomy on a 26-year-old female patient with thyroid cancer. A radical neck dissection with a partial parathyroidectomy and autotransplantation of two parathyroid glands is also completed in the same session. What CPT code(s) should the physician report?

a. 60254, 60500-51, 60512-51
b. 60254
c. 60254, 60512-52
d. 60254, 60500-51, 60512

110. A physician performs a 6 cm midline celiotomy to remove a patient's enlarged spleen by means of cautery. Abdominal exploration was performed, and the lymph nodes surrounding the inferior mesenteric artery that were noted to be abnormal were also removed. What CPT code(s) describes the surgery performed by the physician?

a. 38120, 49000-51
b. 43631
c. 38100, 38999-59
d. 49000, 38102

111. Which form is used to make a patient aware of the potential monetary liability they will have if their procedure is not likely to be covered by Medicare?

a. Advance Beneficiary Notice
b. National Coverage Determination
c. Health Insurance Portability and Accountability Act (HIPAA) Release
d. Payment Plan Contract

112. A gastroenterologist performs a gastric bypass surgery on an obese patient with a body mass index of 52. During the procedure, the size of the stomach is reduced by 77%; the intestine is bypassed from the duodenum and then attached to the ileum. The pylorus is preserved and left intact. Which CPT code best describes the surgery performed?

a. 43842
b. 43843
c. 43845
d. 43847

113. What is the difference between presumptive and definitive testing?

a. Presumptive testing confirms the presence of a drug class; definitive testing identifies the quantity or presence of a drug.
b. Presumptive testing is based on exhibited signs and/or symptoms; definitive testing is based on lab results.
c. Presumptive testing assumes a diagnosis; definitive testing confirms a diagnosis.
d. Presumptive testing requires additional observation time; definitive testing requires a blood draw.

114. Code the following note:

A male patient with a medical history of chronic obstructive pulmonary disease (COPD) presented to the emergency room 3 days ago with tachycardia and shortness of breath. He was intubated and admitted with acute respiratory failure (ARF) due to an acute exacerbation of COPD. Upon follow-up with the patient today, dark sputum was noted in the intubation tube, and testing confirmed aspiration pneumonia. I will start the patient on 875 mg of amoxicillin every 12 hours and follow up tomorrow.

a. 99232, J69.0
b. 99232, J44.1, J96.00, J96.0, R00.0
c. 99231, J69.0, J96.00, J44.1
d. 99233, J96.00, J44.1, J69.0

115. Alzheimer's disease with early onset usually presents itself in which age group?

a. 30–40 years old
b. 40–50 years old
c. 50–60 years old
d. 60–70 years old

116. Which is NOT considered inclusive to hydration services?

a. Catheter declotting
b. Subcutaneous catheter access
c. Flush solution
d. Catheter flush

117. Medical necessity has been established if a laboratory runs additional testing on a urine sample to determine the presence of a drug class that was not in question during confirmation testing.

a. True
b. False

118. A patient is seen in the emergency room with a thermal burn to the left thigh because of a fire. The patient denies feelings of hypothermia. Vitals are obtained, and a physical examination reveals that approximately 4% of the body is affected by second-degree burns, and nonviable tissue needs to be removed to avoid the risk of infection. After consent is obtained, the physician debrides the wound, cleanses the area, and applies a gauze. The patient is discharged and told to follow up with their primary care physician in 2 days. What CPT code(s) should be reported for this encounter?

a. 16020
b. 99283-25, 16020
c. 16020, 99282
d. 99282-25, 16020

119. In the *Current Procedural Terminology* book, how is the icon "Excludes" meant to be interpreted?

    a. It may identify services that are not bundled and may lead the user to a more appropriate code.
    b. A causal relationship should be presumed between the two conditions.
    c. It may include services that are bundled and cannot be separately billed.
    d. An additional code should be reported to fully describe a condition.

120. What is/are the code(s) for the repair of an incarcerated hernia in the inner groin requiring mesh placement on a 32-year-old female patient?

    a. 49507
    b. 49507, 49568
    c. 49553
    d. 49553, 49568

121. A patient has an elective bilateral vasectomy under regional anesthesia. The procedure is completed within 15 minutes. What CPT and ICD-10-CM code(s) should the provider report?

    a. 55250, 89321, Z30.8
    b. 55250, 00921, Z30.2
    c. 55250-50, Z30.8
    d. 55250, Z30.2

122. A patient with preexisting hypertension presents to the office at 23-weeks' gestation for prenatal care. Her blood pressure is slightly elevated, and a transabdominal ultrasound shows the fetus is small for dates. The provider advises rest and to follow up as normal. How would the provider code the visit if the patient has an insurance that accepts the global obstetrical package?

    a. 0502F, 76816, O10.012, Z3A. 23
    b. 99213-25, 76815, O10.012, O36.5910, Z3A. 23
    c. 99213-25, 76816, O10.012, Z3A. 23
    d. 0502F, 76815, O10.012, O36.5910, Z3A. 23

123. Which service is NOT bundled into pediatric critical care CPT 99475?

    a. A blood transfusion is given to a 2-year-old patient with sickle cell disease.
    b. The doctor suspects meningitis on a 4-year-old patient and performs a lumbar puncture to test the fluid around the spinal cord.
    c. A central line is inserted to stabilize a 5-year-old patient in respiratory arrest.
    d. A suprapubic aspiration is performed on a 3-year-old patient who has blood in her urine.

124. ICD-10-CM codes R50.9, R05, R53.81, and J02.9 are all symptoms of J10.00.

    a. True
    b. False

125. What must the documentation for a consultation include?

   a. Which family member prompted the consultation, a written report of the physical findings/ recommendations, and the time spent discussing the recommended treatment plan
   b. The reason for the consultation, the time spent discussing the recommended treatment plan, and a medical decision-making of moderate complexity
   c. Documentation of assumption of care, who requested the consultation, and the consulting providers' professional opinion
   d. Who requested the consultation, the consulting providers' professional opinion, and a written report that is provided to the referring physician

126. A patient has a colonoscopy in which the provider removes three polyps from the transverse colon. The first polyp is removed by means of a hot snare technique, and the following two polyps are removed using hot biopsy forceps. What CPT code(s) should be reported for this encounter?

   a. 45388
   b. 45385, 45384-59, 45384-59
   c. 45385, 45384-59
   d. 45385

127. If a physician administers cyclophosphamide over 154 minutes, irinotecan over 72 minutes, and panitumumab over 15 minutes intravenously to a patient with pancreatic cancer, how should this be reported?

   a. 96413, 96415x3, 96417x2
   b. 96413, 96413-59x2, 96415, 96417
   c. 94613, 96415x2, 96417x2
   d. 96413, 96413-59, 96415x2, 96417

128. A radiation oncologist reviews the port films, dose delivery, and treatment parameters of a 52-year-old female patient who has received external beam therapy three times in the current week. He also spends 15 minutes examining the patient and collecting an intake of her response to the treatment program. Which CPT code(s) should the physician report?

   a. 77435, 99213-25
   b. 77427
   c. 77431
   d. 99213-25, 77401 x 3 units

129. A physician provides a G1P0 39-weeks twin gestational patient with antepartum care, delivery, and postpartum care. Baby A was delivered vaginally without complications, and Baby B was delivered by caesarean due to fetal tachycardia. Assign the correct ICD-10-CM and CPT codes.

   a. 59400, Z37.0 and 59510-51, O36.8392, Z37.0
   b. 59510, O76, Z3A.39, Z37.0 and 59409-51, Z3A.39, Z37.0
   c. 59410, Z37.2 and 59510-51, O76, Z37.2
   d. 59409, Z3A.39, Z37.0 and 59510-51, O76, Z3A.39, Z37.0

130. Code a polyp found in the transverse colon.

    a. D12.3
    b. K51.40
    c. K63.5
    d. D12.6

131. When seen next to a diagnosis code, the term "Excludes 2" indicates that the condition excluded is not part of the condition represented by the code and that the patient may have both conditions simultaneously.

    a. True
    b. False

132. A male patient is admitted with symptoms of a persistent cough and temperature of 101.2. A skin test reveals that the patient has tuberculosis. His medical history is positive for HIV. Assign the appropriate diagnosis codes for this patient.

    a. A18.4, R05, R50.9, B20
    b. A15.9, B20
    c. B20, A15.9
    d. A18.4, Z21

133. If in the assessment, the provider reports diabetes and dermatitis due to oils, which diagnosis code(s) should be reported?

    a. E11.620
    b. E11.69, L24.1
    c. E11.9, L24.1
    d. None of the above—query the provider to clarify which type of diabetes the patient has

134. Which healthcare professional may NOT report medical nutrition therapy?

    a. Endocrinologist
    b. Registered nurse
    c. Dietician
    d. Nutritionist

135. A patient relocates after receiving treatment for an arm fracture. The patient schedules an appointment with a new orthopedist to remove the cast. The orthopedic office should report the fracture diagnosis code with the seventh character A to indicate active treatment.

    a. True
    b. False

136. The physician suspects malignancy and decides to remove two lesions from the patient's back to confirm. The size of the first lesion has a diameter of 0.5 cm, and the excised diameter is 1.0 cm. The size of the second lesion has a diameter of 0.3 cm, and the excised diameter is 1.5 cm. Which CPT code(s) should be reported?

    a. 11600, 11600-51
    b. 11401, 11402-51
    c. 11401, 11402-59
    d. 11402, 11401-59

137. Code the following surgical note:

54-year-old male is experiencing left-sided weakness and visual disturbance. An MRI revealed a lesion in the brain. He presents today for a biopsy. General anesthesia is given, and the area is shaved and cleaned. The brain lab system is synced with prior MRI images to confirm the accurate placement of burr hole drilling. A cutting needle is inserted into the frontal lobe, and lesion location is confirmed with the brain lab system. A portion of the lesion is obtained without complication. All instruments removed, and the incision is sutured.

a. 61140
b. 61750
c. 61751
d. 61575

138. In which scenario would the modifier 52 be appended?

a. An IUD removal is not completed because the patient reports severe pain when the speculum is inserted.
b. The surgeon decides to terminate a coronary balloon angioplasty and stent placement when the patient becomes hypertensive after receiving anesthesia in the hospital operating room.
c. A provider decides to stop a gallbladder removal procedure after the patient has extensive bleeding at the incision site.
d. A patient receives an x-ray of one femur when the doctor ordered bilateral views.

139. Age, gender, height, and race are the four key factors in calculating a person's forced vital lung capacity (FVC). If FVC is calculated to be 3.00 L and anything under 80% is abnormal, what would be the cutoff value to a normal FVC?

a. 3.2 L
b. 2.8 L
c. 2.4 L
d. 2.0 L

140. Code the following note:

44025
A 43-year-old new female patient with a history of type I diabetes was referred to my office by Dr. White, her primary care physician. Patient complains of blurred vision that began 2 weeks ago, however, reports compliance to a strict, healthy diet and to prescribed 10 mg of dexamethasone every day for 1 month. Given that the only change appears to be the dexamethasone, I suspect the blurred vision is an adverse reaction and will decrease the dosage to 5 mg per day. Patient will follow up with me in 1 week if symptoms persist.
Total face-to-face time with the patient was 30 minutes, of which 20 minutes were spent counseling the patient.

a. 99203, H53.8, E10.9
b. 99242, H53.8, T38.0X5A, E10.9
c. 99202, H53.8, E10.69
d. 99243, H53.8 E10.39

141. An 88-year-old patient with Medicare comes in for her yearly flu shot. After receiving a 0.5 mL single shot dose of preservative-free Alfuria intramuscularly, the provider observes the patient for 15 minutes to monitor any adverse reactions. How should the provider code for this encounter?

    a. 90471, 90656, Z23
    b. 99211-25, 90471, 90656, Z23, Z03.89
    c. G0008, 90656, Z23
    d. 96372, 90686, Z23

142. Health behavior assessment and intervention codes capture services related to mental health.

    a. True
    b. False

143. An orthopedic surgeon performs a meniscectomy for a right radial tear using an arthroscope. During the procedure, the surgeon removes a piece of the damaged meniscus from the lateral compartment of the knee and shaves the articular cartilage of the same compartment. A separate incision was made to remove a 6 mm loose body in the medial compartment. The surgery was completed without any complications. What procedure and diagnosis code(s) should be reported?

    a. 29882, 29877-51, 29874-51, S83.203A
    b. 29881, 29874-59, S83.281A
    c. 29887, 29874-59, S83.281A
    d. 29881, 29874-51, S83.203A

144. A 69-year-old patient with a medical history of diabetes is evaluated in the emergency room for a urinary tract infection. After performing a comprehensive history and exam, the physician prescribes 100 mg of Macrobid every 12 hours and admits the patient to observation status to monitor for sepsis. After seeing an improvement in symptoms, the physician discharges the patient the following day. What CPT and ICD-10-CM code(s) should be reported for the entirety of the patient's stay?

    a. 99235, N39.0, B97.89
    b. 99284, 99217, E11.69, N39.0
    c. 99219, 99217, N39.0, E11.9
    d. 99218, 99217, N39.0

145. Consultation codes 99241-99245 have been deemed as not medically necessary and are no longer reimbursed by Medicare. This decision would fall under which term?

    a. Local Coding Determination
    b. National Coding Determination
    c. Carrier Coding Determination
    d. Governed Coding Determination

146. A patient receives a positron emission technology (PET) scan at rest, where a metabolic evaluation study, including ventricular wall motion was performed using PET imaging. A computed tomography (CT) was performed at the same time. What CPT code(s) should the radiologist report?

    a. 78429
    b. 78430
    c. 78429, 76497-59
    d. 78430, 76497-59

147. A urologist performs a laparoscopic adrenalectomy and excises a retroperitoneal mass in the same session. How should this be coded?

    a. 49329
    b. 60545
    c. 60650-22
    d. 60650, 49203-51

148. A patient is in labor with plans to deliver vaginally. An epidural is administered at 17:30. After several hours of pushing, the obstetrician determines that the cervix is swollen, and the baby must be delivered via a c-section. The patient consents, the baby is delivered, and both are discharged to the recovery room at 22:15. What CPT code(s) should the anesthesiologist report?

    a. 01967-23, 01968, 99140
    b. 01967, 01968
    c. 01967, 01968, 99140
    d. 01967-23, 01968

149. What describes a surgical procedure that removes a portion of the vertebral body to relieve pressure on the spinal cord and nerves?

    a. Insertion of interspinous process stabilization device
    b. Corpectomy
    c. Spinal fusion
    d. Laminectomy

150. A patient opts to replace his semi-rigid penile prosthesis with a multicomponent, inflatable penile prosthesis. What CPT code(s) should the urologist report if this was completed in one encounter?

    a. 54415, 54405-51
    b. 54416
    c. 54405, 54415-51
    d. 54405

Answer Key and Explanations

1. D: Minimal, moderate, and deep sedation all allow the patient to undergo a procedure without pain and without being completely unconscious. If a patient receives minimal sedation, they are responsive after receiving verbal stimulation. Moderate sedation causes a patient to respond only after tactile stimulation. General anesthesia causes the patient to be completely unarousable, even with painful stimulation.

2. D: Although CPT code 97530 does describe therapeutic activities, the focus is directed at improving functional performance, whereas the correct CPT code 97110 works to develop range of motion. The CPT code for a soft tissue massage (or manual therapy 97140) is based on 15-minute increments, however, anything over 8 minutes prior to or after can be counted as a unit. Based on this, the 23 minutes spent can be counted as two units. Sequencing is based on highest RVU.

Coding crosswalk for a rotator cuff tear is classified as a muscle strain, so answer B, which specifies "other injury," can be eliminated. Because the patient is in the recovery period of the injury, the seventh character would not be considered active but subsequent.

3. C: A diaphragm resection is reported with CPT codes 39560-39561. The use of a biologic mesh makes the repair complex, whereas a simple repair would implement only internal sutures.

4. C: The documentation supports an expanded problem-focused history with a medical decision-making of low complexity. Therefore, the highest level of service rendered is a 99213. When reporting a routine venipuncture, use CPT code 36415. CPT code 36410(a) is reported when it is medically necessary for the physician to draw a patient's blood, and 36416 describes capillary blood collected through a skin prick—certainly not enough to fill two vials. CPT code 99000 can be used to report a specimen being transported to an outside laboratory, but that is unknown in this scenario. A generic urinalysis is reported with CPT code 81002 unless specifically stated that an automated analyzer (81005), a commercial kit (81007), and/or an agar test (81020) was utilized.

5. A: To code 99203-99205, the provider must document a detailed and/or comprehensive history intake, which must include past medical, family, and social history. For codes 99201-99202, a past medical, family, and social history intake is not required. Answers B and D are for the evaluation of an established patient and are not applicable to this scenario because the patient is new.

6. B: The correct sequencing of the code would be as follows: side effect of the drug, medication that caused the adverse effect, and the underlying condition for why the drug is being taken. In this scenario, because the anemia is caused by a malignancy, ICD-10-CM guidelines state that the malignancy should be the principal diagnosis "followed by the appropriate code for the anemia (such as D63.0, Anemia in neoplastic disease)."

7. B: Although CPT 99211 can be reported for limited assessments performed by nonphysician staff members, the vaccine and allergy history intake is considered vaccine related and not separately reportable. CPT 90460 is reported when a physician provides counseling about the benefits and risks associated with the vaccine and signs and symptoms that would indicate an adverse reaction. Because the physician did not document seeing the patient at this encounter, report CPT 90471 for the administration of the immunization.

8. D: Answers A and B can be eliminated because the complete pulmonary function test includes interpretation of the test results; therefore, the review of this would not be considered separately

127

identifiable. The CPT code 94060 includes spirometry before and after a bronchodilator has been administered, so a separate spirometry code (94010) would be inappropriate. Last, a modifier is not needed because the procedures are routinely done in conjunction with each other.

9. C: Although a foreign body was removed, 57415 in answers A and B cannot be reported because anesthesia was not used. The documentation supports an expanded problem-focused history and moderate-level decision-making, so the appropriate E/M would be a 99213. When comparing answers C and D, bear in mind that ICD-10-CM requires sequencing "the underlying condition first, followed by the manifestation."

10. C: A central nervous system assessment is comprised of multiple screenings that are reported with CPT codes 96105-96146 and includes, but is not limited to, the following elements: use of standardized instruments for staging and rating clinical dementia; evaluation for behavioral symptoms using standardized screening instruments; and development, updating, revision, and/or review of an Advance Care Plan. A review of high-risk medications is also included in the central nervous system assessment; however, if in the same encounter a prescription is issued, the clinician should document and report the treatment with an appropriate E/M.

11. A: 64493 is used for the initial injection of an anesthetic, followed by 64494 and 64495 as add-on codes for the other two levels. Because there are two sides of a facet joint, modifier LT would be amended to show the carrier that the procedure occurred on the left side of the spine.

In answer B, CPT codes 0216T-0218T exclude fluoroscopic guidance and refer the biller to codes 64490-64495.

In general, modifier 59 would not be used on add-on codes, so Answer C can be eliminated.

Answer D describes an injection in the interlaminar epidural or subarachnoid space and is not the correct procedure code for this circumstance.

12. D: When the injury is treated with Steri-Strips or bandages, it should be reported with an E/M code and not a procedure code. The E/M is a 99213 because the history of the visit is expanded problem focused, the exam is problem focused, and the medical decision-making is low. A suicide attempt would not be coded because the documentation is not specific as to whether the lacerations were an attempt at suicide.

13. D: To report an esophagogastroduodenoscopy, see CPT code range 43235-43259. In this scenario, the procedure is not considered diagnostic (43235) because the physician is stating the patient has GERD. Additionally, the tissue sample was obtained by means of biopsy forceps and not by brushing or washing. The secondary procedure is a reflux test and an esophageal pH test by means of a bravo capsule, which evaluates the level of acid refluxing into the esophagus. Although CPT 91035 doesn't specifically state a capsule in the description of the code, it would fall under a "mucosal attached" placement. A nasal catheter was not used, so reporting CPT 91034 would be incorrect.

14. B: The first procedure documented is a bronchoscopy, reported with CPT codes 31622-31654. Because the procedure was specifically aimed at confirming a diagnosis based off a previously confirmed malignancy, the bronchoscopy would be considered diagnostic (CPT 31622). The second procedure performed is a mediastinotomy with removal of cancerous tissue. An incision made into the parasternal intercostal space is considered transthoracic, making the correct procedure code 39010. Sequencing is based off the highest RVU value, and modifier 51 is appended to the bronchoscopy procedure code to indicate that multiple procedures were performed in the same session.

15. B: The patient is having the colonoscopy done because they have been experiencing symptoms. Therefore, the colonoscopy would be considered diagnostic versus screening. CPT crosswalk for a diagnostic colonoscopy is 45378. The documentation gives no indication that any bleeding was identified and controlled. When the surgeon performing the primary procedure is simultaneously administering anesthesia services, modifier 47 is appended rather than billing an additional anesthesia delivery code.

16. B: Although CPT codes 10021, 10041, and 60100 all represent percutaneous procedures, only CPT 60100 describes the use of a large bore needle to obtain a specimen. When multiple biopsies are taken from the same nodule, only report CPT 60100 once. If a separate nodule is biopsied, report 60100 a second time with modifier 59, indicating a procedure on a sperate anatomical site.

17. A: CPT defines an initial nursing facility service (NFS) as "the first encounter with the patient by the admitting physician to nursing facilities." Although the patient can be evaluated and treated by other medical staff in the meantime, only the physician responsible for the admission may report the initial comprehensive visit (99304-99306). If other medical personnel do provide treatment, those visits would be reported using the subsequent nursing facility care encounter codes (99307-99310). When selecting the level of service, bear in mind that all three components (history, exam, and medical decision-making) are required. Although the physician did complete a comprehensive history and examination of the patient, consider that the patient's condition is established and improving and that prescription drug management puts the level of risk at moderate. This makes the level of complexity for the visit low and brings the encounter down to CPT 99304.

18. C: Magnetic resonance imaging (MRI) uses magnets, radio waves, and a computer to display detailed pictures of the inside of the body. Tomography uses waves of energy to create three-dimensional, computer-generated images of any internal structure. Computed tomography is cross-sectional images of the body obtained by a narrow beam of x-rays that quickly rotates around the body.

19. A: CPT code 88331 is used to report only a single specimen. In this scenario, there are two separate specimens being sent to the pathologist. The first specimen, with one frozen section, is reported with CPT code 88331. The second specimen has two tissue blocks with frozen sections, thus represented by coding 88331 for the first tissue block, followed by 88332 for the additional tissue block. CPT code 88329 is inclusive to 88331 and should not be reported separately.

20. B: CPT guidelines define critical care as an illness or injury that acutely impairs one or more vital organ systems, where there is a high probability of imminent or life-threatening deterioration in the patient's condition. Additionally, to report a critical care service, the documentation should provide evidence of high-complexity medical decision-making (e.g., endotracheal tube insertion, defibrillation, fluid administration for shock, Narcan, etc.).

Answer B is the only option listed that contains documentation to support critical care services. This male patient has two life-threatening conditions, in which emergent intervention is provided to prevent further deterioration. In answer A, the female patient may have a life-threatening condition; however, administering oxygen via a nasal cannula and/or transfusing blood does not qualify as critical care. Management of a patient who receives chronic ventilator therapy is also not considered critical care because the medical decision-making involved in the therapy is quite low. The care a patient receives after having surgery would be considered routine and postoperative, regardless of where they are sent, unless a complication arises in which one or more of the vital organ systems begins to deteriorate in a fashion that poses a threat to life.

21. B: The statement is false. According to CPT, a new patient is one who has "not received professional services from the physician." In lieu of this, because the cardiologist only interpreted an electrocardiogram and did not actually provide care to the patient, a new patient E/M service should be billed.

22. C: In this case, the patient is not at risk, and most organs either are not developed and/or cannot be visualized in the first trimester. Thus, this would constitute as waste due to the provider overutilizing services that result in unnecessary cost. AAPC defines fraud as purposely billing "for services that were never given or to bill for a service that has a higher reimbursement than the service provided." Abuse is payment for services "that are billed by mistake by providers."

23. A: The statement is true. When it comes to reporting anesthesia services, qualifying circumstances are factors that put a patient at an unusually high health risk. A qualifying circumstance is reported with CPT codes 99100-99140, which are listed separately, in addition to the primary anesthesia code. If reporting one of these add-on codes, documentation must be submitted to support the necessity of such services.

24. D: The CPT codes for cytopathology smears are dependent on the payer and the method used to test the specimen. HCPC II G0148 does accurately describe the test method; however, this code is used for Medicare payers only. As the documentation does not specify that this is the case, it should be assumed that the carrier is non-Medicare. The appropriate non-Medicare CPT for this test method is 88175. CPT 88141 is always reported as a secondary code for the associated physician interpretation. Regarding the diagnosis, the primary ICD-10-CM code should be synonymous with the reason for the encounter, which in this scenario would be the gynecological exam (Z01.419). Although Z12.4 does describe a screening of the cervix, it specifically is excluded from the diagnosis list "when the screening is part of general gynecological examination (Z01.4-Z01.42)." Any abnormal findings are reported as secondary and/or tertiary.

25. D: Surgical procedures on the nervous system are identified by where inside the skull they occur. A meningioma is being excised from above the tentorium cerebelli, otherwise known as supratentorial (CPT 61512). The removal of an extradural hematoma is inclusive to the primary craniectomy code because the finding is incidental and the same surgical site is used for its removal. If the surgeon had to create a separate incision to access the extradural hematoma, that excision could be reported separately with modifier 59.

26. C: The physician performed a detailed examination and the medical decision-making was moderate in complexity due to the new problem and the issuance of a prescription drug. Because the patient has already been receiving care in a hospital setting for 3 days, the visit would be considered subsequent hospital care, making the level of inpatient service a 99232 and eliminating answers B and D.

A burn caused by a chemical would be considered a corrosion because it is not caused by heat, electricity, and/or radiation, thus eliminating the remaining choice of A. Additionally, when multiple burns on the same anatomic location and laterality are being treated, identify and code only the highest degree of burn recorded in the diagnosis. In this case, only the third-degree burns on the right hand and the second-degree burns on the left hand would be reported. Although the skin infection is a sequela, the seventh character in the corrosion code would remain "A" and sequenced first to indicate that the patient is still receiving active treatment for the reason of admission.

27. A: The eight elements included in the history of present illness are: location, quality, severity, duration, timing, context, modifying factors, and associated signs and symptoms.

28. D: An E/M is always billed when a patient is seen in the emergency department because it is unscheduled and urgent. In this case, the documentation encompasses an expanded problem-focused history, a comprehensive evaluation, and low-level decision-making. These three components lead the coder to 99282. Modifier 57 is appended to indicate that the decision for surgery was made just prior to the procedure and is not bundled. CPT coding crosswalk confirms that a closed treatment of a dislocated elbow is CPT code 24600. Application of a splint is represented by CPT code 29105 but is not applicable when performed with a surgery to correct the dislocation. ICD-10-CM crosswalk for dislocation of left elbow is S53.105A.

29. A: The code for a joint fusion using a posterior approach is 22612. In this scenario, there are three fusion levels: L2-L3, L3-L4, and L4-L5. Following the primary code, 22614 would be billed twice and with no modifier because it is an add-on code. ICD-10-CM code M51.37 is for degenerative discs in the lumbosacral region; however, L2-L5 is considered the lumbar region.

30. D: 0484T describes a transcatheter mitral valve replacement via a thoracic approach. CPT code 33430 describes a mitral valve replacement in which cardiopulmonary bypass is initiated. CPT code 0483T describes a transcatheter mitral valve replacement with a percutaneous approach; however, the documentation identifies a transthoracic incision. Catheterization is bundled into the procedure and is not separately identifiable unless the provider documents extenuating circumstances (i.e., no prior study available, inadequate visualization, etc.).

31. B: When a patient is receiving hospice care, Medicare will not reimburse the physician for services rendered that are unrelated to the terminal illness unless submitted with modifier GW. In Answers C and D, a separate, identifiable E/M is not to be billed because the procedure is considered minor (1- to 10-day global period) and includes an inherent E/M component.

32. D: The diagnosis is always based on the provider's documentation, which in this case would be obesity. Coding guidelines also state that if there is a reportable diagnosis related to weight, "the BMI can be assigned from documentation of someone other than the patient's provider, such as nursing notes."

33. D: A goiter is an abnormal enlargement of the thyroid gland. The removal of that gland is a thyroidectomy, represented by CPT codes 60240-60271. CPT 60270 is selected based on the approach used. CPT codes 21602 and 32900 are obtained by using the coding crosswalk for resection of the chest wall and describe the removal of a tumor and one or more ribs. CPT 32140 is a thoracotomy, which involves pulling apart the ribs to reach and remove a lung cyst.

34. A: Per CPT guidelines, administration of contrast materials is given through the following routes: intravascular, intra-articular, and intrathecal. Alternate routes also include orally and/or rectally; however, the "contrast administration alone does not qualify as a study 'with contrast.'"

35. A: The statement is true. In general, modifier 50 is not appended on cystourethroscopies because human anatomy has only one bladder. However, if the descriptor includes "with ureteral catherization," the procedure can be performed twice and billed once with modifier 50 because there are two ureters. CPT 52000 does not include this descriptor.

36. C: CPT crosswalk for anesthesia administered during a total knee replacement is 01402. Although CPT 01991 does describe a nerve block, it is considered monitored anesthesia care because the patient is awake. However, in this scenario, general anesthesia is being used for the primary procedure, and the femoral nerve block is administered for postoperative pain management. Therefore, the nerve block would be billed as CPT 64447 with modifier 59 to indicate that it is separately reportable from the primary procedure. If, on the other hand, the nerve block was being used as a component of the general anesthesia, CPT 64447 would be considered inclusive to the general anesthesia and not reported separately. Ultrasound guidance is not currently bundled with the administration of a nerve block and, when used, should be reported separately with CPT 76942.

37. A: After receiving deoxygenated blood from the body through the vena cava, the right atrium pumps blood into the right ventricle. The right ventricle sends the blood to the lungs to be oxygenated. The left atrium receives blood from the lungs through the pulmonary veins and pumps it into the left ventricle via the mitral valve. The left ventricle then distributes oxygenated blood to tissues throughout the body.

38. B: The left coronary artery and the right common carotid artery would each be considered their own vascular family. Therefore, when the starting point of selective catheterization is the aorta, the left coronary artery would be considered first order (36215) in the vascular family and the right common carotid artery would be considered the second order (36216). Modifier 59 is appended to indicate that a different vascular family was examined in one session. Contrast materials and catheterization into the aorta are inclusive to the two procedures and are not to be separately coded.

39. A: CPR is not a bundled service to critical care and should be reported separately with CPT code 92950.

40. B: The CPT code 11201 is an add-on code and would not receive a modifier. Local anesthesia is included in the primary procedure code and would not be reported separately with CPT 00300.

41. C: Pain while urinating (R30.9) is a symptom of a urinary tract infection (N39.0), and a sore throat (R07.0) and fever (R50.9) are symptoms of acute tonsillitis caused by bacteria (J03.8, B95.3). Neither of these three codes should be reported because ICD-10-CM guidelines stipulate that when a definitive diagnosis is present, signs and/or symptoms should not be additionally listed on the claim.

42. C: The code description "tube thoracostomy" is not clearly stated in the documentation, but CPT crosswalk for a "tube placement" followed by "chest" leads the coder to CPT 32551. CPT 32550 describes the insertion of a catheter that allows the patient to drain pleural fluid in an outpatient setting. Moderate sedation can be separately billed but only by the provider administering the medication. The J93 series is circumstantial (e.g., spontaneous, acute). Even though the term "recurrent" is not used, it does describe the background of the patient's condition and so would fall into the other specified diagnosis rather than unspecified.

43. B: The statement is false. Time-based coding can be done only when the documentation supports that at least 50% of the time was spent counseling and/or coordinating the care of the patient.

44. A: The role of the kidneys is to filter blood before it is transported back to the heart, remove waste materials from food and medication, and regulate blood pressure by excreting excess sodium. The ureters propel urine from the kidneys into the bladder.

45. A: Because the reason for the visit was a routine colonoscopy, the "encounter for screening for malignant neoplasm of colon" (Z12.11) would be the first-listed code. ICD-10-CM guidelines advise that if there is a finding during a screening, the finding may be used as an additional code. In this example, the colon polyp (K63.5) is a physical finding and would be listed as the secondary diagnosis.

46. D: Osteopathic manipulation services do not include evaluation and management services. Although the patient's treatment has already been established, the osteopathic physician has enough supporting documentation to report a separate evaluation and management code. Manipulation services rendered by an osteopathic physician are reported with CPT codes 98925-98929. A chiropractor would report manipulative treatment to two body regions with CPT 98940, and a physical therapist would report CPT 97140.

47. D: CPT codes 90935-90937 require the presence of a physician. If a physician visits the patient prior to or after the dialysis treatment but does not document their presence during the hemodialysis services, bill only the appropriate evaluation and management code (CPT 99232). Additionally, unless otherwise stated, diagnosis selection should reflect the causal relationship that exists between hypertension and ESRD (I12.-, N18.-)—they should not be reported as unrelated. ICD-10-CM Z99.2 is appended to indicate hemodialysis status.

48. A: When a wound is repaired with a tissue adhesive, Medicare accepts only the HCPC code G0168. Answers B and C accurately reflect the repair code for a commercial carrier. An E/M would not be added as an additional charge because the patient's encounter was only for the repair, thus eliminating answer D.

49. A: The statement is true. Regardless of how a sternal closure is performed, it would be considered integral to this, and any other open cardiac procedure, when a sternal approach is used as the method of exposure. If a sternal closure were performed as the only procedure to repair an injury, the closure would then be reported.

50. C: A "gaping" injury and/or "single-layer closure" is indicative of an intermediate repair and a "superficial" injury and/or use of a "tissue adhesive" is indicative of a simple repair. Because the repairs are not in the same classification, each repair is reported in a single code, sequenced from the most to the least severe (eliminating answers B and D), with modifier 59 appended to the less complicated procedure(s). Local anesthesia is included in these procedures, as is debridement unless the provider specifically indicates that it is extensive. In answer A, an HCPC's code for tissue adhesive would be reported only if the patient had Medicare.

51. D: Modifier 26, indicating only a professional component of the study, would be inappropriate because the radiologist who obtained the images and interpreted the results works for the clinic that owns the x-ray machines. By reporting the procedure without a modifier, the clinic is requesting 100% reimbursement of the study, which includes the technical and professional components. When searching the index in the ICD-10-CM book, a stress fracture is related to fatigue and is coded as a bone disorder as opposed to an injury.

52. D: CPT 98960 is used by nonphysician healthcare professionals who provide education to patients that enable them to self-manage established conditions. CPT 99078 could also be used to report lactation services, but these are specifically rendered in a group setting. CPT 98966 is used for healthcare management via the telephone, and CPT 99211 is not considered the most appropriate descriptor for services rendered in this instance.

53. D: A urodynamics study is a diagnostic test to evaluate the function of the bladder. When performed using calibrated equipment, it becomes known as a complex cystometrogram (51726-51729). In CPT code 51728, a complex cystometrogram is performed in conjunction with voiding pressure studies. In the provider's documentation, the bladder is filled with water, and voiding times and volume are recorded, thus fulfilling the requirements for this code. CPT code 51726 in answers A and B only describe a complex cystometrogram without the voiding pressure studies. Electromyography (EMG) studies were performed without a needle to evaluate pelvic floor activity and are represented by 51784. An intraabdominal voiding pressure study (51797) can be inferred in that the provider had earlier inserted a rectal catheter and, after instructing the patient to cough, obtained an abdominal pressure measurement. A complex urinary flow study (51741) was performed in obtaining the maximum urinary flow rate through calibrated equipment. This procedure is missing in answers B and C. Modifier TC (indicating only a technical component) is amended on all the procedures because the provider is not interpreting the results to the patient. Modifiers 51 and/or 59 is not amended on any procedure (A and B) because these are routinely billed together.

54. D: NCCI stands for National Correct Coding Initiative and was created by CMS to prevent unbundling and prevent incorrect payments. Column one represents a correct code when listed next to column two. There are three edits listed with the combination of the two columns: 0, 1, and 9. Edit 0 means that the two codes should never, under any circumstance, be reported together. Edit 1 means that the procedures may be coded together with the use of a modifier. Edit 9 means that the edit does not apply.

55. D: The upper respiratory tract consists of the nose, nasal cavity, pharynx, and larynx. The lower respiratory tract includes the trachea, primary bronchi, lungs, and the bronchioles and alveoli within the lungs.

56. B: It would not be appropriate to add modifier 52 to 80053 in answer A. In answer C, 80051 and 80053 would not be reported together because CPT guidelines state that "when two or more panel codes include the same tests, report the panel with the highest number of tests in common." Because the glucose test is not included in 80051, 82947 would be added to 80051, with no modifier 59, because the procedures are routinely billed together, thus eliminating answer D.

57. B: The "application of casts and strapping" guidelines located in the surgery section of the CPT book explain that a splint is reported when the physician providing the initial service does not perform, or expects to perform, any other treatment. In this case, because the visit was minimal and directed only at the sprain with no intended follow-up care, only the application of the splint would be reported. The application itself is considered static because the wrist is completely immobilized. HCPC crosswalk for a wrist splint, in addition to knowing the difference between static and dynamic, would immediately lend itself to the correct HCPC: S8451.

58. D: An open appendectomy procedure is reported with CPT 44950. A metastatic colon malignancy is a cancer that began in the colon but has spread to other areas. In this scenario, that means that the primary malignancy is the colon, and the secondary malignancy is the appendix. Additionally, ICD-10-CM guidelines state that when "treatment is directed toward the metastatic site only, the metastatic site is designated as the principal/first-listed diagnosis. The primary malignancy is coded as an additional code." The malignancy codes do not specifically state "appendix," but the ICD-10-CM coding crosswalk in the neoplasm table assigns this diagnosis as C78.5 secondary malignant neoplasm of large intestine and rectum.

59. A: The primary role of the tonsils is to remove bacteria that enter though the oral and nasal cavity. Antigens are molecules located on the surface of pathogens and trigger the formation of antibodies. Lymph nodes filter lymph and form lymphocytes. B cells secrete antibodies that assist in destroying bacterium causing disease.

60. D: To calculate the total number of units, it is important to understand that anesthesia time is measured in 15-minute intervals (or in fractions thereof). In this scenario, take the total number of minutes spent on the procedure (105) and divide it by 15. The total number of time units is 7. The time units are then added to the base unit (10) for a total of 17 units.

61. B: To bill a comprehensive electrophysiologic evaluation (93619-93622), the following five components must be documented: right atrial pacing (93610), right atrial recording (93602), right ventricular pacing (93612), right ventricular recording (93603), and bundle-of-His recording (93600). If the documentation does not support all five components, each study must be reported separately, as opposed to billing the procedure with a "reduced services" modifier. The exception to this rule would be if an add-on procedure were performed and required to be reported in addition to the comprehensive electrophysiologic evaluation. In this case, however, the attempted induction arrhythmia (93618) is not an add-on code and can be reported in addition to the primary procedures.

62. A: The statement is true. G codes apply to various healthcare screenings. If a patient is experiencing any symptoms that initiate the encounter, it then becomes diagnostic, and an appropriate CPT code would be selected instead.

63. C: An intractable migraine is one that is continuous and obstinate to conventional treatment. If a migraine is preceded by symptoms of vision disturbances and/or transient muscle weakness, those symptoms are collectively known as aura. A migraine with aura is also called a classical migraine. Status migrainosus describes a severe, debilitating migraine that lasts longer than 72 hours and usually results in hospitalization.

64. D: A level II HCPC code describes medical devices, supplies, medication, and/or other services that a provider and/or entity used during a service provided to a patient. Advanced life support (ALS) fits this description because it is a set of life-saving protocols administered in transit. Radiation treatment management and a diagnostic colonoscopy describe a level I HCPC code, otherwise known as a CPT code. If the patient was asymptomatic and the colonoscopy was for screening purposes only, a level II HCPC code could be assigned. However, a diagnostic procedure implies a past medical/family history that puts the patient at risk and/or symptoms that warrant the procedure. A malignant neoplasm describes an ICD-10-CM code because it is a diagnosis.

65. B: CPT code 93304 describes an echocardiography used to evaluate a congenital defect. In this case, the provider is screening for any trauma-related injuries to the heart. Bearing in mind that the study is limited leads you to CPT 93308. Modifier 26 is used on all CPT codes because the procedures are being performed in a hospital setting. Therefore, only the professional component of the service should be billed. Modifier TC is reported by the entity providing the equipment, which in this case would be the hospital. Modifier 59 is not necessary because the procedures are routinely done in conjunction with each other.

66. B: When choosing between CPT 51840 and 51841, consider that obesity reduces the operative field, increases surgical time, and poses difficulties in surgical technique. It is therefore considered one of several complicating factors to this surgery because it has an abdominal approach.

Additionally, although the obesity is not the reason for the surgical encounter, it nevertheless should be coded due to the impact it has on the procedure.

67. B: A gastroscopy is a procedure that uses an endoscope to examine the stomach and some parts of the intestinal tract. An endoscopy uses a thin tube through a natural opening in the body to examine the digestive tract. A laparotomy is a large incision in the belly to gain access into the abdominal cavity.

68. D: An adenoidectomy and a tonsillectomy were performed in this surgical encounter (the root word –ectomy literally means the surgical removal of an anatomical structure). The adenoidectomy was done first and, if coded alone, would fall under one of two categories: primary (CPT 42830-42831) or secondary (CPT 42835-42836). A primary adenoidectomy refers to the initial removal of the adenoid, whereas a secondary adenoidectomy occurs when adenoid tissue that was once removed has grown back. Because the documentation states that "the adenoid tissue . . . regrew after the initial adenoidectomy," a coder can infer that this procedure is secondary. However, distinguishing between the two procedures is not necessary when done in conjunction with a tonsillectomy because the procedures are bundled into two nonspecific CPT codes (42820 and 42821). Billing for an adenoidectomy and a tonsillectomy separately, as shown in answers A and C, is considered unbundling and is not allowed under the Correct Coding Initiative (CCI) edits. Regarding the sequencing of the diagnoses, ICD-10-CM guidelines state that when two conditions meet the definition for principal diagnosis, either can be sequenced first. In this scenario, J35.2 or G47.33 could have been first listed because the procedures were to resolve both conditions in the same encounter.

69. A: CPT surgery guidelines uphold that local infiltration, metacarpal/metatarsal/digital block, or topical anesthesia is always included in the surgical package. Under monitored anesthesia care (MAC), a patient is sedated but typically still aware, and the presence of qualified anesthesia personnel is required. Spinal and regional anesthesia is used for a variety of different procedures and is also separately reportable.

70. D: Toxic adenoma E05.2- is a thyroid nodule that may secrete hormones into the body that results in an overactive thyroid. Graves' disease E05.0- is an autoimmune disorder that attacks the thyroid, resulting in overactivity. Hashimoto's disease E06.3 is also an autoimmune disorder; however, it usually results in an underactive thyroid. Acosta disease T70.29- is altitude sickness. Even if a coder is unfamiliar with these terms, by locating the ICD-10-CM code that correlates to the condition, a coder can infer which body system a diagnosis relates to.

71. C: The procedure performed was a mediastinotomy with a biopsy, represented by CPT 39000. CPT code 39401 is reported for a mediastinoscopy, which is the insertion of a scope through an incision in the notch above the sternum. ICD-10-CM crosswalk for a mass found on the chest wall is R22.-. Although the approach is cervical, the location of the mass is mediastinal, falling under the anatomical site of the trunk.

72. B: All observation codes (99234-99236) include a comprehensive history and exam. The medical decision-making of this condition is considered high (number of diagnoses and risk of complication), making the CPT 99236. Even though pneumonia is the reason for admission, ICD-10-CM guidelines stipulate that a confirmed HIV diagnosis takes precedence in sequencing when the reason for admission is HIV related.

73. A: CPT 76815 is a limited ultrasound, in which only the fetal heartbeat, position, placental location, and/or volume of amniotic fluid are evaluated. In this scenario, much more was done than a limited study. The ultrasound technician documented age-appropriate fetal measurements, which are supported by CPT 76816. A biophysical profile (BPP) was also done, which monitors the fetus's movements, tone, and breathing as well as evaluates the volume of amniotic fluid. Each of these elements counts as 2 units of grading to evaluate the general well-being of the fetus. The desired score of a BPP is 8/8. Because a fetal nonstress test (NST) was completed in conjunction with a BPP, report CPT 76818 instead of CPT 76819. Modifier TC is used to reflect that only a technical component of the procedure was completed. However, because the patient received these services in an obstetrical office that employs the physicians providing prenatal care and owns the ultrasound equipment, the code should be submitted without modifiers TC or 26 to receive 100% reimbursement.

74. A: Modifier 76 is used to identify a repeated procedure, but the test was performed on a separate fetus. Modifier 22 indicates increased procedural services; however, the services were not increased. Rather, a separate, identifiable test was rendered, and the modifier 59 would therefore apply to the second fetal nonstress test.

75. D: Understanding immunology and antibody results are imperative to proper code selection and to be able to support any necessary repeat testing. Antibody isotypes IgM assist in attacking infectious pathogens and are indicative of an acute infection. Antibody isotypes IgG are formed as an infection subsides and help the body fight against future attacks from the same bacteria. When the results show IgG positive, it indicates immunity. When a patient has an infection, the results will show IgM positive, but as the IgG antibodies haven't fully formed yet to provide the body with immunity, that result will come back negative.

76. C: A circumcision procedure includes a local anesthetic, also known as a ring block. Therefore, an additional anesthesia code (CPT 64450) should not be reported as a secondary code, nor should modifier 52 be appended on the primary procedure. The code notes for ICD-10-CM code Z41.2 specifically state that this diagnosis should be used only when the procedure is elective and not related to a specific diagnosis. In this case, because the procedure is related to a recurring condition the patient is experiencing, the infection should be the primary diagnosis. The diagnosis crosswalk would be "infection" followed by "penis," which directs the coder to N48.29.

77. C: To determine which services to report for this encounter, it is important to understand which services were rendered on the last. The patient had an open biopsy of the axillary lymph nodes (CPT 38525) last week. This procedure has a postoperative 90-day global period. This means that any related services provided to the patient within that time are reported with zero-charge CPT 99024. Services such as biopsy results, follow-up incisional care, and any postoperative complications are all inclusive to this code. As the patient was given biopsy results, CPT 99024 should be reported for this encounter. However, CPT guidelines also state that when it comes to diagnostic procedures, "care of the condition for which the diagnostic procedure was performed . . . is not included and may be listed separately." In this case, that care begins with the discussion of treatment options, which is reported by means of E/M CPT 99212. Modifier 24 is appended to indicate that is it unrelated to postoperative care, and modifier 25 is appended to indicate it is separately identifiable to CPT 99024. ICD-10-CM crosswalk for lymphoma, diffuse large cell, is C83.34.

78. A: Epinephrine is listed in alphabetical order in the HCPC book under "Table of Common Drugs." The documentation reflects a dosage of 0.3 mg, so three units of 0.1 mg epinephrine (J0171) should be reported. The injection of the medication is reported with CPT code 96372 and includes an inherent E/M component unless the provider goes beyond the normal assessment of the patient prior and/or after administration of a drug.

79. D: Per ICD-10-CM, a sequela describes "complications or conditions that arise as a direct result of a condition." In this case, the chronic pain would be a condition that resulted from a prior injury. Removal of a foreign body is active treatment of a laceration. Removal of a fixation device and prescription drug management are both considered routine and subsequent care.

80. B: When a hematology procedure that could be billed alone is encompassed in another code, only the most complex of the two should be reported. Because CPT 85046 includes the reticulocyte count, billing CPT 85044 as secondary despite using a different method would be considered an unbundling of services. Per ICD-10-CM guidelines, an organ or tissue transplant status code is for use "only if there are no complications or malfunctions of the organ or tissue replaced." As the testing is to determine whether the engraftment was successful, a bone marrow transplant status code would not be appropriate until deemed by the provider.

81. A: When splitting/providing relief in the middle of a procedure, the anesthesiologist who provides services for the longest amount of time bills for the anesthesia services in their entirety. In this scenario, Anesthesiologist Z provided 60 minutes more than Anesthesiologist A and so would bill for the entire 4.5 hours. Even though Anesthesiologist A provided 1.75 hours, they would not submit any coding to the insurance carrier.

82. A: The statement is true. An insurance carrier will use these three measures to determine what the RVU of a procedure should be. Then, based on that, a medical coder can determine what the expected payment should be. Generally, the higher the RVU of a procedure is, the higher the payment will be.

83. A: When deciding between a routine extracapsular cataract removal and a complex extracapsular cataract removal, bear in mind the code descriptor for a complex procedure involves "devices or techniques not generally used in a routine cataract surgery (e.g., iris expansion device)." Because iris hooks were used, the procedure is complex (CPT 66982). When it comes to the diagnosis, do not get confused with the anatomy of the eye. Although the cornea works with the lens to help refract light, they are anatomically separate, thus eliminating answer B as an acceptable choice. A congenital condition is one that is genetic and/or present from birth. The documentation does not specify the origin, nor does it indicate when the lens abnormality began. Symptoms of a cataract include clouded and discolored lenses but should not be reported unless the physician clearly identifies this as the diagnosis. Coding crosswalk for diseases of the lens leads a coder to H27.8 (other specified disorders of lens).

84. D: The hepatitis B surface antigen test was not performed, so the actual panel code in answer A was not completed, leaving each test to be reported separately. It would not be appropriate to add modifier 52 to 80074 in answer B. Because the provider did not specify which side the lower abdominal pain was on, it would be reported as unspecified with R10.30, eliminating answer C.

85. C: HIPAA is in place to reduce the level of risk associated with a potential violation and/or breach. In answer C, even though a breach has occurred, the hospital has appropriate preventative measures in place and is not in violation of HIPAA. Leaving a laptop in an unattended vehicle or medical records outside is high-risk behavior that gives opportunity for an unauthorized person to access protected health information (PHI) and/or electronic protected health. In answer D, a medical practice is required to perform a risk analysis to PHI and/or ePHI and rectify any failures within a timely manner.

86. C: When coding a telehealth encounter for an outpatient practice that occurs over audio-video technology (e.g., Skype), the appropriate office visit E/M would be reported with modifier 95. The patient must initiate the telehealth encounter. Although similar, CPT code 99442 is billed when a patient initiates communication with a provider through an online patient portal. ICD-10-CM Z20.828 is reported only when a patient does not exhibit any symptoms of a disease the patient is suspected to have been exposed to.

87. C: Two of the highest three components should be used to determine the level of complexity. In this case, because the complexity of data and level of risk were moderate, the MDM is considered moderate. If the highest two components fall into different categories, the lower of the two would determine the score. This scoring method is the same for both the 1995 and the 1997 documentation guidelines.

88. B: The statement is false. CPT 00520 is anesthesia services for closed-chest procedures. However, a thoracotomy is an open procedure involving a surgical incision to the chest wall. The correct CPT code that should be reported is 00540 (anesthesia for thoracotomy procedures involving lungs, pleura, diaphragm, and mediastinum).

89. B: Modifier 78 represents an additional, unplanned surgery during the global period for a complication arising for the initial procedure. In this case, the complication would be the infection. Modifier 58 is generally used when a secondary procedure is planned prior to or during the time of the initial procedure. Modifier 79 is used to indicate two unrelated procedures. Modifier 25 is for use on E/M codes only.

90. A: Observation hospital care is provided to patients who are not sick enough to be admitted. Therefore, it is considered an outpatient service and is covered under Medicare part B.

91. B: The treatment of flu-like symptoms is considered a non-obstetric service, and a separate E/M can be billed for reimbursement. All other answer choices would be included in the global obstetrical package as routine care.

92. B: The underlying condition should always be first listed, which in this case would be the SARS-CoV-2 infection (U07.1). The description of the code then prompts the biller to list the manifestations, which would be the unspecified bronchitis (J40). In answer A, cough would not be coded as a symptom because the patient's illness is confirmed. Answers C and D, which include a suspected exposure code, can also be eliminated because this code is used only when the existence of the illness in the patient is unknown or negative.

93. C: Anesthesia time begins when the provider begins to prepare the patient for anesthesia services. This usually will take place in the operating room or an equivalent area. Although answer B would not be incorrect as a chosen starting point, answer C is more accurate according to the anesthesia time definition. Preoperative evaluations of the patient, such as a history intake, cannot be counted as anesthesia time.

94. C: The CPT crosswalk for x-ray of knee directs the coder to 73560-73580. Because two views were obtained, the correct code would be 73560 (radiologic examination, knee; 1 or 2 views). Modifier TC and modifier 26 indicate only technical and professional components; however, because the x-ray was performed in a physician's office, 73560 would be reported without either because the practice provided both components. In terms of diagnosis, the knee pain would not be reported because it is a symptom of a definitive diagnosis.

95. B: The statement is false. Per ICD-10-CM, "Results must be documented in the report for each of the elements described in the code description." If the provider does not document a given element, they must include a reason for non-visualization for the CPT to be reported.

96. D: Acute trauma results from a single incident, whereas chronic trauma is repeated, usually over the course of months or years. In this scenario, the documentation does not specify, so the coder should assume acute trauma. There is no mention of obstruction, so ICD-10-CM code selection is K44.9, followed by the cause of the hernia. When an exam shows evidence of abuse, the abuse is no longer considered suspected but confirmed.

97. D: CPT code 77067 is a screening mammogram. In this case, the mammogram would be diagnostic because the purpose is to rule out and/or make a diagnosis based on physical exam findings. Code 77065-50 is an inappropriate use of the modifier because there exists a bilateral procedure code. A breast lump should only be coded to "mass" and not as a neoplasm unless specifically stated in the diagnosis. When deciphering the location of the mass, 12 o'clock is at the top of each breast, and the point of movement is clockwise. Therefore, 4 o'clock in the right breast is equivalent to the lower-inner quadrant, and 6 o'clock in the left breast is in the middle of the two lower quadrants.

98. D: Durable medical equipment is represented by E codes, orthotic procedures are L codes, and enteral therapy is inclusive to B codes in the HCPC manual.

99. D: The diaphragm separates the thoracic cavity from the abdominal cavity by means of skeletal muscle. When the diaphragm contracts, air is drawn into the lungs. It therefore plays a key role in respiration. The mediastinum is surrounded by loose connective tissue and contains several anatomical structures including the heart. Connective tissue is distributed throughout the body to form tendons, ligaments, cartilage, and fat.

100. B: The physical status modifiers are used to identify different levels of complexity associated with the patient's condition. Additionally, they provide information surrounding the circumstances of the anesthesia service and are a useful tool to support medical necessity. Modifier P3 describes a patient with a severe systemic disease, such as uncontrolled diabetes and/or hypertension. Multiple organ dysfunction is reported with modifier P5, which describes a patient who is not expected to survive without an operation. A recent myocardial infarction and sepsis both describe a severe systemic disease that is a threat to life and is reported with modifier P4.

101. D: If 99402 is part of a more complex service, it would not be separately identifiable, thus eliminating answer A. Because 99385 includes counseling/anticipatory guidance/risk factor reduction interventions, the additional 30 minutes that the provider spent discussing contraceptives would not be considered a significant, separately identifiable E/M service, eliminating answer B. Last, because time is not a factor when selecting a preventative service, 99355 reflected in answer C, indicating a prolonged service would not apply.

102. A: The statement is true. When multiple endoscopic procedures are performed in the same session, only the most extensive service should be reported. In this case, it would be the surgical endoscopy because it has a higher revenue value.

103. C: Regarding Z08, ICD-10-CM guidelines state: "The follow-up codes are used to explain continuing surveillance following completed treatment of a disease. [...] They imply that the condition has been fully treated and no longer exists." When using a follow-up code as the primary reason for an encounter, a history code indicating what condition the patient originally had should be assigned as secondary. Aftercare codes are used to describe the continued treatment of a disease. In this case, the malignancy has been eradicated, the disease no longer exists, and aspirin is being used merely as a preventative measure. History codes can never be reported as first listed; rather, a follow-up code or other current disease and/or condition should precede it.

104. C: A clinical pathology consultation was rendered at the request of the primary care physician. The consultation is considered limited as opposed to comprehensive because it was done without the review of the patient's history and medical records. E/M codes can be billed only when a patient is physically evaluated by the provider. In this case, the pathologist only evaluated a specimen.

105. B: Place of service (POS) codes "specify the entity where service(s) were rendered." In this case, hospice care was provided in an office, which would correspond to POS 11. POS 34 is hospice care provided in a facility, POS 71 is a public health clinic that provides ambulatory medical care, and POS 62 is an outpatient rehabilitation facility providing services that would include physical and occupational therapy.

106. B: Photodynamic therapy applies a photosensitizing agent by either an external or endoscopic application. An external application is applied directly onto a patient's lesions, whereas an endoscopic application is an injection into the bloodstream, where it is absorbed by cells all over the body. Based on this differentiation, the documentation supports only an endoscopic application. The code notes for CPT 96570 and 96571 indicate they are add-on codes to the bronchoscopy procedure, which is represented by CPT 31641. Any drug administration is inclusive to photodynamic therapy, making CPT 96409 not separately billable.

107. C: It is common practice to perform both an electrophysiology (EP) study and a cardiac ablation procedure in the same session. These procedures have been bundled in the CPC manual, and the coding of such is dependent on the type of arrhythmia being treated. The EP study and cardiac ablation are not to be reported separately. In this scenario, the patient has atrial fibrillation, which is reported with CPT 93656. When fluoroscopy is used for guidance rather than for diagnostic imaging, it is usually not reported separately from the primary procedure. Moderate sedation can be reported when used, and selection is based on time. CPT 99152 and 99153 are counted in 15-minute intervals. When the procedure does not fall on a 15-minute interval, it must at least meet the halfway point of the time stated to be reported.

108. A: The primary diagnosis on an inpatient record would be the primary reason the patient was admitted. In this case, because a definitive diagnosis could not be confirmed, the symptom of chest pain would be selected instead. The previously confirmed chronic conditions would also be coded because they affect the management of inpatient care. Diabetes would be coded to an unspecified code because the term "with" implies a causal relationship between the conditions that is not implicitly documented. Per ICD-10-CM guidelines, a rule-out code is not assigned when "any signs or symptoms related to the suspected condition are present."

109. C: The CPT code for a thyroidectomy with a radical neck dissection is 60254 and sequenced first because it is the primary procedure with the highest RVU. CPT 60500, which describes a parathyroidectomy, is bundled into a thyroidectomy. Therefore, the two procedures should never be reported together. Parathyroid autotransplantation (CPT 60512) involves the removal of all four parathyroid glands. If not all four glands are removed, report the code with modifier 52 to indicate reduced services. As this is an add-on code, do not append modifier 51.

110. C: CPT 38120 is the removal of the spleen by means of a laparoscope. The physician performed a midline celiotomy (an abdominal incision), which is an open procedure, eliminating this option. CPT 43631 describes the removal of certain portions of the stomach and was not the procedure performed. An exploratory laparotomy (or abdominal exploration) is inclusive to a splenectomy procedure and should not be reported separately. Additionally, CPT 38102 is reported when the spleen is involved in an extensive disease such as malignancy. On the other hand, CPT

38100 fully describes the open splenectomy, and CPT 38999 is used for the removal of mesenteric lymph nodes because there is no specific code for this procedure.

111. A: National Coverage Determination is a reference guide for physicians to determine which services are covered by Medicare. The HIPAA Release is a form that must be signed by the patient prior to release of medical records and can be revoked at any time. The HIPAA Privacy Rule is in place to protect the patient's health information.

112. C: In this scenario, the gastroenterologist performed a procedure known as a biliopancreatic diversion with duodenal switch (BPD/DS). A BPD/DS removes a portion of the stomach and transfers parts of the duodenum and small intestine to the lower end of the large intestine in an effort to limit intestinal absorption for weight loss. CPT codes 43842-43843 describe gastric restrictive procedures without gastric bypass. However, gastric bypass was done in rearranging the small intestine to connect to the ileum.

113. A: A presumptive test reports whether the patient is positive or negative for a specific drug. A definitive test would analyze which specific agent and/or how much of that agent is in the patient's system.

114. D: When a history intake is unattainable due to the patient's condition, the documentation should clearly reflect the circumstances involved in their admission. When done appropriately, the history of present illness (HPI), review of systems (ROS), and medical, social, and family history can be credited toward the level of service. This documentation supports a detailed history (HPI, ROS, and medical history) and decision-making of high complexity (new problem with additional workup and acute illnesses that pose a threat to life), making CPT 99233 the most accurate description of services rendered. Regarding selection and sequencing of the diagnoses, always select the reason for the admission as the primary diagnosis code. In this case, the patient was admitted for ARF (J96.00). The secondary code would be the underlying COPD (J44.1), and conditions arising after admission would be tertiary and so forth. Tachycardia would not be reported because it is a symptom of ARF and symptoms are not reportable when the underlying disease has been confirmed.

115. B: According to CPT, the rarest form of Alzheimer's disease occurs before 30 years of age. Early onset Alzheimer's disease usually affects those between the age of 40 and 50 years old. The most common form of Alzheimer's disease occurs after the age of 65 and is largely contributed to a combination of environmental and genetic factors.

116. A: Catheter access, standard supplies such as a flush solution, and the flush at the end of the infusion are all considered necessary to facilitate the infusion and are inclusive to CPT codes 96360-96361. Declotting a catheter involves the injection of a thrombolytic agent to dissolve the clot and is separately reportable with CPT 36593.

117. B: The statement is false. To establish medical necessity, the provider/laboratory must indicate the drug class they are screening for prior to the test.

118. B: When billing for physician services in the emergency room, it is appropriate to report a standalone E/M when the documentation supports its necessity in determining the need for appropriate treatment. Modifier 25 is necessary to the E/M code when being billed alongside a procedure and/or surgery to indicate a separately billable service. In this case, the documentation supports an expanded problem-focused history intake and exam and a decision-making of moderate complexity. CPT code 99283 meets these criteria, whereas CPT code 99282 reflects a medical decision-making of low complexity and does not accurately portray the services rendered.

The emergency room visit is always the first listed code, followed by the procedure and/or surgery performed.

119. A: The "Excludes" note identifies services that are not bundled into a procedure and may be reported in addition to the primary code. It may also lead the user to another code that would be more appropriate for the procedure being reported. Answer B describes "with." Answer C describes the icon "Includes." Answer D describes the "code also" note attached to a diagnosis.

120. A: There are several different types of hernias that are categorized by their location. A hernia located in the inner groin is inguinal, and a hernia located on the outer groin is femoral. The repair of an incarcerated inguinal hernia on a 32-year-old patient is coded to CPT 49507. Hernia mesh is used to reduce the risk of recurrence, and implantation of it is inclusive to an inguinal, umbilical, femoral, and laparoscopic hernia repair.

121. D: A vasectomy includes a sperm analysis and regional anesthesia and should not be unbundled for higher reimbursement. A vasectomy includes both unilateral and bilateral sides, so modifier 50 should never be appended. In this circumstance, CPT 55250 should be billed as a standalone procedure to encompass all services delivered. Additionally, although the documentation does not give a specific diagnosis, it can be inferred from "elective" that the procedure is not to treat an underlying illness or injury. Therefore, Z30.2 (encounter for sterilization) is the evident diagnosis for this type of procedure because the patient is being sterilized. Z30.8 (encounter for other contraceptive management) can be used for an encounter discussing post vasectomy sperm count.

122. A: The global obstetrical package includes routine prenatal care visits and blood pressure checks, so a placeholder code (0500F-0503F) is used to report that a visit occurred instead of an E/M code. CPT 76816 is reported when biometric measurements are taken of the fetus, whereas CPT 76815 is limited to one element of the fetus, such as the position or heartbeat. Per ICD-10-CM, codes beginning with O35- and O36- are reported only "when the fetal condition is actually responsible for modifying the management of the mother."

123. C: A blood transfusion (CPT 36430, 36440), lumbar puncture (CPT (62270), and suprapubic aspiration (CPT 51100) are all considered inclusive to pediatric critical care services rendered on patients between the age of 2 and 5 years old. A complete list of all additional services can be found in the CPT Section Guidelines for Newborn and Pediatric Services. A central line insertion (CPT 36556) is not bundled into critical care services and may be reported separately.

124. A: The statement is true. In general, R codes are descriptive of a patient's signs and symptoms. ICD-10-CM crosswalk for an unspecified sore throat is J02.9 (acute pharyngitis) and is also considered a symptom of the influenza and pneumonia. Being that there is a definitive diagnosis of an influenza, these symptoms would not be reported to an insurance carrier with J10.00.

125. D: Per CPT guidelines, the Office of Inspector General, and Medicare, a consultation must include who requested the consultation, the consulting provider's professional opinion, and a written report of the findings, which is provided to the referring physician. Time can be used to select the level of E/M; however, it is not required if all three components of the documentation are met (history, exam, and medical decision-making). Additionally, once the provider assumes care, a subsequent code appropriate for that place of service would be reported (e.g., 99211-99215) and not a consultation code.

126. C: When coding colonoscopies, remember that the number of removal techniques is what has a bearing on code selection and not the number of lesions and/or polyps that are being removed. In this case, two techniques are being used: 1) the snare technique (CPT 45385) and 2) the hot biopsy forceps technique (CPT 45384). Modifier 59 is appended onto the secondary code to indicate that separate polyps were removed by two different techniques. CPT 45388 is reported when a provider uses any methods other than snare and hot biopsy forceps to remove a lesion and/or polyp.

127. C: Unless a separate IV site is established for a secondary or tertiary administration, CPT 96413 should be reported only once to represent the initial drug infusion. In this case, it is the cyclophosphamide. The remaining 94 minutes are reported with two units of add-on CPT 96415, which may be reported if the time spent beyond the first hour is between 31 and 60 minutes. CPT 96417 is reported only once per subsequent infusion of a different drug up to the first hour. Consequently, the 72 minutes of irinotecan is reported with a single unit of CPT 96417, and the 15 minutes of panitumumab is also reported with one unit of that same CPT code.

128. B: Treatment management of a patient undergoing radiation therapy is reimbursed by reporting CPT codes 77427-77470. Treatment management includes a review of the port films, dosimetry, dose delivery, treatment parameters, a physical examination, and related counseling. It would therefore not be appropriate to bill for a separate evaluation and management. CPT 77435 describes treatment management for a course of stereotactic body radiation therapy (SBRT), which the patient is not receiving. CPT 77401 describes the actual radiation and not the evaluation from the physician. CPT 77431 is reported when the entire course of therapy consists of one or two treatment sessions; however, a coder can infer from the documentation that the patient in this scenario has or will receive multiple sessions over the course of one or more weeks. Additionally, CPT guidelines advise that only three treatment sessions must occur to support the face-to-face encounter described in CPT 77427.

129. B: The Cesarean delivery (59510) would be sequenced first because this code has the highest RVU and would include the antepartum and postpartum care. The vaginal delivery by itself (59409), without antepartum and postpartum care, would be reported secondary because the charges for the antepartum and postpartum care of the mother have already been included in the Cesarean delivery code.

130. C: Coding crosswalk for a colon polyp would direct the coder to the benign neoplasm table. However, careful examination of the guidelines reveals that if the documentation does not specifically state that a polyp was adenomatous and/or benign, or that a polyp was inflammatory, the most appropriate choice selection would be a code from K63.

131. A: The statement is true. The term "Excludes 2" shows that two seemingly related conditions can be billed in the same encounter. See Section 1 of the Coding Guidelines in the ICD-10-CM 2020 edition for reference.

132. C: Tuberculosis (TB) can usually spread from the lungs to another site via the bloodstream. Because the documentation does not specify whether the TB is primary or secondary, the coder would default to A15.9, as TB unspecified. A cough and fever are symptoms of an underlying illness and would not be coded because a definitive diagnosis of TB is present. Because TB is an HIV-related illness, B20 would be the first listed code.

133. C: When the documentation does not specify which type of diabetes is present, always default to type II. Although there is a causal relationship assumed between diabetes and dermatitis, the documentation reflects that the dermatitis is due to oils, not diabetes. Because the manifestation of dermatitis is not associated with the diabetes, the correct code would be E11.9: diabetes type II without complications.

134. A: Medical nutrition therapy describes nutritional assessments and interventions in a face-to-face or group patient setting and is reported with CPT codes 97802-97804. These codes are used by nonphysician healthcare professionals only. When a physician provides nutritional advice, a preventative service or evaluation and management code should be reported.

135. B: The statement is false. When a patient is in the healing and/or recovery phase of an injury, the seventh character would be D to indicate that the care is subsequent—whether the provider has treated the patient in the past or not.

136. D: Without a pathology report to confirm malignancy, the excision code assumes that the lesion is benign. Code selection is based on the excision size, not the size of the lesion, and the more complex code takes priority in sequence, eliminating answer C. Answers A and B can be incorrect choices due to CPT guidelines outlining that when coding more than one excision, the appropriate modifier would be 59 on each additional procedure.

137. C: The coding crosswalk for a brain biopsy leads to three CPT codes. CPT code 61140 is a burr hole through which a lesion in the brain can be located and biopsied. CPT code 61750 is a biopsy using a CT or MRI scanning technique to locate the lesion in the brain. CPT code 61751 is the same as 61750, with the addition of the use of CT or MRI scanning during the procedure to confirm the location of lesion and/or accurate placement of surgical instruments. In this case, that occurred with the brain lab system. CPT code 61575 is a biopsy done on a different anatomic location and does not describe this procedure.

138. C: Modifier 52 is used to indicate that a procedure was terminated by the provider after anesthesia was given due to extenuating circumstances that affected the health of the patient. Although option B is similar, the surgery specifically was done in the hospital setting, in which case modifier 73 would be appended.

139. C: A forced vital capacity test is the maximum amount of air that can be exhaled from the lungs and is used to determine whether there is an obstruction in the lungs.

To calculate the abnormality, take 0.8 (80%), and multiply it by 3.00 (liters). Anything less than 2.4 L would be considered an abnormal result in this scenario.

140. A: When choosing between an outpatient evaluation and management code or a consultation service code, bear in mind the following four elements: request, reason, report, and intent. Although the first three elements are documented and support a consultation service, the endocrinologist is assuming immediate care of the patient's condition. In this case, the visit is not a consultation but a new transfer of care, which is represented by CPT codes 99201-99205. For this visit, coding based on time would be more advantageous because the history intake and exam appear to be limited. When coding based on time, the provider must document that at least half of the time spent face-to-face with the patient was used to counsel and coordinate care. The provider documented just that, making the appropriate billable code 99203, in which 30 minutes are typically spent with the patient.

The documentation reflects that the blurry vision is most likely due to the dexamethasone; therefore, a causal relationship is not assumed between the two conditions and should not be coded as such. Because an adverse reaction is suspected and not confirmed, it should not be coded. This general rule does not apply to inpatient encounters.

141. C: The patient has Medicare insurance and therefore requires the use of an HCPC code (G0008) in place of a CPT intramuscular injection code. The use of an E/M code in answer B is not warranted because the provider only administered services related to the vaccination. The appropriate diagnosis code for any vaccination would be Z23.

142. B: The statement is false. Health behavior assessment and intervention codes capture services related to a patient's physical health and can be used only when the patient has a physical health diagnosis as the primary reason for treatment—not a mental disorder. Although assessing factors related to the patient's mental state, it is done to promote functional improvement and lessen any obstacles to a patient's recovery.

143. B: The procedures performed on this encounter were the meniscectomy (removal of damaged meniscus from the lateral compartment) with a chondroplasty (shaving of articular cartilage, 29881) and loose body removal by means of an arthroscopy (29874). Because the removal of loose bodies is considered inclusive to the primary procedure, modifier 59 is appended as opposed to modifier 51 to indicate that it was a distinct procedural service due to the separate incision. Answers A and D can be eliminated based on the diagnosis chosen. S83.203A indicates the location of meniscus is unspecified: however, the surgeon removed the damaged meniscus from the lateral compartment, leading the biller to S83.281A.

144. C: When a patient is admitted into observation status from the emergency room, only the observation code is reported for that day. When observation extends past the initial date of service, the initial treatment would be reported with CPT codes 99218-99220. In this scenario, the appropriate level of service would be a 99219, based on the comprehensive history, exam, and moderate decision-making, which can be based off the number of diagnoses and the management option. Discharge from observation on a separate date is reported with CPT code 99217.

Because the diabetes is documented and is a coexisting chronic condition during the time of the encounter, it should follow the reason for admission. Due to a lack of specificity in the diabetes diagnosis, a causal relationship with a UTI is not presumed, and E11.69 should not be coded.

145. B: Decisions regarding coverage are made through evidence-based processes and public opinion. National Coding Determination (NCD) is specific to Medicare coverage nationwide, whereas Local Coding Determination (LDC) is contractor and commercial specific. Carrier and Governed Coding Determinations do not exist.

146. A: PET scans are reported using CPT codes 78429-78434. The documentation specifies that a metabolic study was performed versus a perfusion study, thus eliminating answers B and D. A CT scan is included in the description of CPT 78429, thus making it unable to be separately reportable.

147. C: CPT 60650 describes a laparoscopic adrenalectomy with a biopsy but not the complete removal of a retroperitoneal mass. In contrast, adding modifier 22 indicates increased work and complexity and can be used because there is no CPT to describe a laparoscopic retroperitoneal mass resection. CPT 49329 represents an unlisted laparoscopy procedure that can be used to describe the removal of a retroperitoneal mass but would have to be used in conjunction with CPT 60650 to describe the adrenalectomy procedure. CPT 60545 describes an adrenalectomy with excision of a retroperitoneal mass by means of an abdominal or posterior incision. CPT 49203 also does not describe the procedure because it involves an open excision of an intra-abdominal tumor.

148. D: For a planned vaginal delivery with the use of an epidural, followed by a Cesarean delivery, the correct CPT codes are 10967 followed by add-on code 01968. CPT code 99140 is an add-on code portraying that the procedure was an emergency and that the patient and/or baby has a significant increase in the threat to life. The documentation gives no indication that these services were emergent. Modifier 23 is reported for unusual anesthesia services. This would include—but is

146

not limited to—the use of general anesthesia for a procedure that usually requires only a local anesthetic or none and/or a procedure extending more than 4 hours. In this case, the total procedure time was 4.75 hours, and modifier 23 is appended on the primary procedure code only.

149. B: The insertion of an interspinous process stabilization device is done to increase the space within the neural foramen, release nerve pressure that causes physical pain, and create spinal stabilization. A spinal fusion is a surgical procedure that permanently joins two or more vertebrae into one solid bone so that no space exists between them. A laminectomy is a surgical procedure that removes the lamina to enlarge the spinal canal and relieve pressure on the spinal cord and/or nerves.

150. D: Penile prosthesis procedure codes are based on the type of prosthesis being used. In this scenario, a semi-rigid prosthesis is being replaced by a multicomponent inflatable one. Currently, there are no CPT codes that encompass the removal of one type of prosthesis and insertion of another type. The most common course of action might be to code the removal and insertion separately and amend a multi-procedural modifier on the secondary code. However, CPT 54415 indicates that the prosthesis removed was not replaced by another, which is an inaccurate description of services rendered. In this case, only the insertion (CPT 54405) should be reported because it has the highest RVU value.

How to Overcome Test Anxiety

Just the thought of taking a test is enough to make most people a little nervous. A test is an important event that can have a long-term impact on your future, so it's important to take it seriously and it's natural to feel anxious about performing well. But just because anxiety is normal, that doesn't mean that it's helpful in test taking, or that you should simply accept it as part of your life. Anxiety can have a variety of effects. These effects can be mild, like making you feel slightly nervous, or severe, like blocking your ability to focus or remember even a simple detail.

If you experience test anxiety—whether severe or mild—it's important to know how to beat it. To discover this, first you need to understand what causes test anxiety.

Causes of Test Anxiety

While we often think of anxiety as an uncontrollable emotional state, it can actually be caused by simple, practical things. One of the most common causes of test anxiety is that a person does not feel adequately prepared for their test. This feeling can be the result of many different issues such as poor study habits or lack of organization, but the most common culprit is time management. Starting to study too late, failing to organize your study time to cover all of the material, or being distracted while you study will mean that you're not well prepared for the test. This may lead to cramming the night before, which will cause you to be physically and mentally exhausted for the test. Poor time management also contributes to feelings of stress, fear, and hopelessness as you realize you are not well prepared but don't know what to do about it.

Other times, test anxiety is not related to your preparation for the test but comes from unresolved fear. This may be a past failure on a test, or poor performance on tests in general. It may come from comparing yourself to others who seem to be performing better or from the stress of living up to expectations. Anxiety may be driven by fears of the future—how failure on this test would affect your educational and career goals. These fears are often completely irrational, but they can still negatively impact your test performance.

> **Review Video: 3 Reasons You Have Test Anxiety**
> Visit mometrix.com/academy and enter code: 428468

Elements of Test Anxiety

As mentioned earlier, test anxiety is considered to be an emotional state, but it has physical and mental components as well. Sometimes you may not even realize that you are suffering from test anxiety until you notice the physical symptoms. These can include trembling hands, rapid heartbeat, sweating, nausea, and tense muscles. Extreme anxiety may lead to fainting or vomiting. Obviously, any of these symptoms can have a negative impact on testing. It is important to recognize them as soon as they begin to occur so that you can address the problem before it damages your performance.

> **Review Video: 3 Ways to Tell You Have Test Anxiety**
> Visit mometrix.com/academy and enter code: 927847

The mental components of test anxiety include trouble focusing and inability to remember learned information. During a test, your mind is on high alert, which can help you recall information and stay focused for an extended period of time. However, anxiety interferes with your mind's natural processes, causing you to blank out, even on the questions you know well. The strain of testing during anxiety makes it difficult to stay focused, especially on a test that may take several hours. Extreme anxiety can take a huge mental toll, making it difficult not only to recall test information but even to understand the test questions or pull your thoughts together.

> **Review Video: How Test Anxiety Affects Memory**
> Visit mometrix.com/academy and enter code: 609003

Effects of Test Anxiety

Test anxiety is like a disease—if left untreated, it will get progressively worse. Anxiety leads to poor performance, and this reinforces the feelings of fear and failure, which in turn lead to poor performances on subsequent tests. It can grow from a mild nervousness to a crippling condition. If allowed to progress, test anxiety can have a big impact on your schooling, and consequently on your future.

Test anxiety can spread to other parts of your life. Anxiety on tests can become anxiety in any stressful situation, and blanking on a test can turn into panicking in a job situation. But fortunately, you don't have to let anxiety rule your testing and determine your grades. There are a number of relatively simple steps you can take to move past anxiety and function normally on a test and in the rest of life.

> **Review Video: How Test Anxiety Impacts Your Grades**
> Visit mometrix.com/academy and enter code: 939819

Physical Steps for Beating Test Anxiety

While test anxiety is a serious problem, the good news is that it can be overcome. It doesn't have to control your ability to think and remember information. While it may take time, you can begin taking steps today to beat anxiety.

Just as your first hint that you may be struggling with anxiety comes from the physical symptoms, the first step to treating it is also physical. Rest is crucial for having a clear, strong mind. If you are tired, it is much easier to give in to anxiety. But if you establish good sleep habits, your body and mind will be ready to perform optimally, without the strain of exhaustion. Additionally, sleeping well helps you to retain information better, so you're more likely to recall the answers when you see the test questions.

Getting good sleep means more than going to bed on time. It's important to allow your brain time to relax. Take study breaks from time to time so it doesn't get overworked, and don't study right before bed. Take time to rest your mind before trying to rest your body, or you may find it difficult to fall asleep.

> **Review Video: The Importance of Sleep for Your Brain**
> Visit mometrix.com/academy and enter code: 319338

Along with sleep, other aspects of physical health are important in preparing for a test. Good nutrition is vital for good brain function. Sugary foods and drinks may give a burst of energy but this burst is followed by a crash, both physically and emotionally. Instead, fuel your body with protein and vitamin-rich foods.

Also, drink plenty of water. Dehydration can lead to headaches and exhaustion, especially if your brain is already under stress from the rigors of the test. Particularly if your test is a long one, drink water during the breaks. And if possible, take an energy-boosting snack to eat between sections.

> **Review Video: How Diet Can Affect your Mood**
> Visit mometrix.com/academy and enter code: 624317

Along with sleep and diet, a third important part of physical health is exercise. Maintaining a steady workout schedule is helpful, but even taking 5-minute study breaks to walk can help get your blood pumping faster and clear your head. Exercise also releases endorphins, which contribute to a positive feeling and can help combat test anxiety.

When you nurture your physical health, you are also contributing to your mental health. If your body is healthy, your mind is much more likely to be healthy as well. So take time to rest, nourish your body with healthy food and water, and get moving as much as possible. Taking these physical steps will make you stronger and more able to take the mental steps necessary to overcome test anxiety.

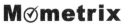

Mental Steps for Beating Test Anxiety

Working on the mental side of test anxiety can be more challenging, but as with the physical side, there are clear steps you can take to overcome it. As mentioned earlier, test anxiety often stems from lack of preparation, so the obvious solution is to prepare for the test. Effective studying may be the most important weapon you have for beating test anxiety, but you can and should employ several other mental tools to combat fear.

First, boost your confidence by reminding yourself of past success—tests or projects that you aced. If you're putting as much effort into preparing for this test as you did for those, there's no reason you should expect to fail here. Work hard to prepare; then trust your preparation.

Second, surround yourself with encouraging people. It can be helpful to find a study group, but be sure that the people you're around will encourage a positive attitude. If you spend time with others who are anxious or cynical, this will only contribute to your own anxiety. Look for others who are motivated to study hard from a desire to succeed, not from a fear of failure.

Third, reward yourself. A test is physically and mentally tiring, even without anxiety, and it can be helpful to have something to look forward to. Plan an activity following the test, regardless of the outcome, such as going to a movie or getting ice cream.

When you are taking the test, if you find yourself beginning to feel anxious, remind yourself that you know the material. Visualize successfully completing the test. Then take a few deep, relaxing breaths and return to it. Work through the questions carefully but with confidence, knowing that you are capable of succeeding.

Developing a healthy mental approach to test taking will also aid in other areas of life. Test anxiety affects more than just the actual test—it can be damaging to your mental health and even contribute to depression. It's important to beat test anxiety before it becomes a problem for more than testing.

> **Review Video: Test Anxiety and Depression**
> Visit mometrix.com/academy and enter code: 904704

Study Strategy

Being prepared for the test is necessary to combat anxiety, but what does being prepared look like? You may study for hours on end and still not feel prepared. What you need is a strategy for test prep. The next few pages outline our recommended steps to help you plan out and conquer the challenge of preparation.

STEP 1: SCOPE OUT THE TEST

Learn everything you can about the format (multiple choice, essay, etc.) and what will be on the test. Gather any study materials, course outlines, or sample exams that may be available. Not only will this help you to prepare, but knowing what to expect can help to alleviate test anxiety.

STEP 2: MAP OUT THE MATERIAL

Look through the textbook or study guide and make note of how many chapters or sections it has. Then divide these over the time you have. For example, if a book has 15 chapters and you have five days to study, you need to cover three chapters each day. Even better, if you have the time, leave an extra day at the end for overall review after you have gone through the material in depth.

If time is limited, you may need to prioritize the material. Look through it and make note of which sections you think you already have a good grasp on, and which need review. While you are studying, skim quickly through the familiar sections and take more time on the challenging parts. Write out your plan so you don't get lost as you go. Having a written plan also helps you feel more in control of the study, so anxiety is less likely to arise from feeling overwhelmed at the amount to cover.

STEP 3: GATHER YOUR TOOLS

Decide what study method works best for you. Do you prefer to highlight in the book as you study and then go back over the highlighted portions? Or do you type out notes of the important information? Or is it helpful to make flashcards that you can carry with you? Assemble the pens, index cards, highlighters, post-it notes, and any other materials you may need so you won't be distracted by getting up to find things while you study.

If you're having a hard time retaining the information or organizing your notes, experiment with different methods. For example, try color-coding by subject with colored pens, highlighters, or post-it notes. If you learn better by hearing, try recording yourself reading your notes so you can listen while in the car, working out, or simply sitting at your desk. Ask a friend to quiz you from your flashcards, or try teaching someone the material to solidify it in your mind.

STEP 4: CREATE YOUR ENVIRONMENT

It's important to avoid distractions while you study. This includes both the obvious distractions like visitors and the subtle distractions like an uncomfortable chair (or a too-comfortable couch that makes you want to fall asleep). Set up the best study environment possible: good lighting and a comfortable work area. If background music helps you focus, you may want to turn it on, but otherwise keep the room quiet. If you are using a computer to take notes, be sure you don't have any other windows open, especially applications like social media, games, or anything else that could distract you. Silence your phone and turn off notifications. Be sure to keep water close by so you stay hydrated while you study (but avoid unhealthy drinks and snacks).

Also, take into account the best time of day to study. Are you freshest first thing in the morning? Try to set aside some time then to work through the material. Is your mind clearer in the afternoon or evening? Schedule your study session then. Another method is to study at the same time of day that you will take the test, so that your brain gets used to working on the material at that time and will be ready to focus at test time.

STEP 5: STUDY!

Once you have done all the study preparation, it's time to settle into the actual studying. Sit down, take a few moments to settle your mind so you can focus, and begin to follow your study plan. Don't give in to distractions or let yourself procrastinate. This is your time to prepare so you'll be ready to fearlessly approach the test. Make the most of the time and stay focused.

Of course, you don't want to burn out. If you study too long you may find that you're not retaining the information very well. Take regular study breaks. For example, taking five minutes out of every hour to walk briskly, breathing deeply and swinging your arms, can help your mind stay fresh.

As you get to the end of each chapter or section, it's a good idea to do a quick review. Remind yourself of what you learned and work on any difficult parts. When you feel that you've mastered the material, move on to the next part. At the end of your study session, briefly skim through your notes again.

But while review is helpful, cramming last minute is NOT. If at all possible, work ahead so that you won't need to fit all your study into the last day. Cramming overloads your brain with more information than it can process and retain, and your tired mind may struggle to recall even previously learned information when it is overwhelmed with last-minute study. Also, the urgent nature of cramming and the stress placed on your brain contribute to anxiety. You'll be more likely to go to the test feeling unprepared and having trouble thinking clearly.

So don't cram, and don't stay up late before the test, even just to review your notes at a leisurely pace. Your brain needs rest more than it needs to go over the information again. In fact, plan to finish your studies by noon or early afternoon the day before the test. Give your brain the rest of the day to relax or focus on other things, and get a good night's sleep. Then you will be fresh for the test and better able to recall what you've studied.

STEP 6: TAKE A PRACTICE TEST

Many courses offer sample tests, either online or in the study materials. This is an excellent resource to check whether you have mastered the material, as well as to prepare for the test format and environment.

Check the test format ahead of time: the number of questions, the type (multiple choice, free response, etc.), and the time limit. Then create a plan for working through them. For example, if you have 30 minutes to take a 60-question test, your limit is 30 seconds per question. Spend less time on the questions you know well so that you can take more time on the difficult ones.

If you have time to take several practice tests, take the first one open book, with no time limit. Work through the questions at your own pace and make sure you fully understand them. Gradually work up to taking a test under test conditions: sit at a desk with all study materials put away and set a timer. Pace yourself to make sure you finish the test with time to spare and go back to check your answers if you have time.

After each test, check your answers. On the questions you missed, be sure you understand why you missed them. Did you misread the question (tests can use tricky wording)? Did you forget the information? Or was it something you hadn't learned? Go back and study any shaky areas that the practice tests reveal.

Taking these tests not only helps with your grade, but also aids in combating test anxiety. If you're already used to the test conditions, you're less likely to worry about it, and working through tests until you're scoring well gives you a confidence boost. Go through the practice tests until you feel comfortable, and then you can go into the test knowing that you're ready for it.

Test Tips

On test day, you should be confident, knowing that you've prepared well and are ready to answer the questions. But aside from preparation, there are several test day strategies you can employ to maximize your performance.

First, as stated before, get a good night's sleep the night before the test (and for several nights before that, if possible). Go into the test with a fresh, alert mind rather than staying up late to study.

Try not to change too much about your normal routine on the day of the test. It's important to eat a nutritious breakfast, but if you normally don't eat breakfast at all, consider eating just a protein bar. If you're a coffee drinker, go ahead and have your normal coffee. Just make sure you time it so that the caffeine doesn't wear off right in the middle of your test. Avoid sugary beverages, and drink enough water to stay hydrated but not so much that you need a restroom break 10 minutes into the test. If your test isn't first thing in the morning, consider going for a walk or doing a light workout before the test to get your blood flowing.

Allow yourself enough time to get ready, and leave for the test with plenty of time to spare so you won't have the anxiety of scrambling to arrive in time. Another reason to be early is to select a good seat. It's helpful to sit away from doors and windows, which can be distracting. Find a good seat, get out your supplies, and settle your mind before the test begins.

When the test begins, start by going over the instructions carefully, even if you already know what to expect. Make sure you avoid any careless mistakes by following the directions.

Then begin working through the questions, pacing yourself as you've practiced. If you're not sure on an answer, don't spend too much time on it, and don't let it shake your confidence. Either skip it and come back later, or eliminate as many wrong answers as possible and guess among the remaining ones. Don't dwell on these questions as you continue—put them out of your mind and focus on what lies ahead.

Be sure to read all of the answer choices, even if you're sure the first one is the right answer. Sometimes you'll find a better one if you keep reading. But don't second-guess yourself if you do immediately know the answer. Your gut instinct is usually right. Don't let test anxiety rob you of the information you know.

If you have time at the end of the test (and if the test format allows), go back and review your answers. Be cautious about changing any, since your first instinct tends to be correct, but make sure you didn't misread any of the questions or accidentally mark the wrong answer choice. Look over any you skipped and make an educated guess.

At the end, leave the test feeling confident. You've done your best, so don't waste time worrying about your performance or wishing you could change anything. Instead, celebrate the successful

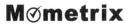

completion of this test. And finally, use this test to learn how to deal with anxiety even better next time.

> **Review Video: <u>5 Tips to Beat Test Anxiety</u>**
> Visit mometrix.com/academy and enter code: 570656

Important Qualification

Not all anxiety is created equal. If your test anxiety is causing major issues in your life beyond the classroom or testing center, or if you are experiencing troubling physical symptoms related to your anxiety, it may be a sign of a serious physiological or psychological condition. If this sounds like your situation, we strongly encourage you to seek professional help.

Tell Us Your Story

We at Mometrix would like to extend our heartfelt thanks to you for letting us be a part of your journey. It is an honor to serve people from all walks of life, people like you, who are committed to building the best future they can for themselves.

We know that each person's situation is unique. But we also know that, whether you are a young student or a mother of four, you care about working to make your own life and the lives of those around you better.

That's why we want to hear your story.

We want to know why you're taking this test. We want to know about the trials you've gone through to get here. And we want to know about the successes you've experienced after taking and passing your test.

In addition to your story, which can be an inspiration both to us and to others, we value your feedback. We want to know both what you loved about our book and what you think we can improve on.

The team at Mometrix would be absolutely thrilled to hear from you! So please, send us an email at tellusyourstory@mometrix.com or visit us at mometrix.com/tellusyourstory.php and let's stay in touch.

Additional Bonus Material

Due to our efforts to try to keep this book to a manageable length, we've created a link that will give you access to all of your additional bonus material:

mometrix.com/bonus948/cpc

157

Made in the USA
Monee, IL
12 December 2022

21255951R00092